# CONTENTS

CHURCHILL'S POCKETBOOK OF

# Clinical

*For Churchill Livingstone*:

*Publisher*: Timothy Horne
*Project manager*: Ninette Premdas
*Project editor*: Jim Killgore
*Editor*: Kathleen Orr
*Design*: Erik Bigland
*Project controller*: Nancy Arnott

# CHURCHILL'S POCKETBOOK OF
# Clinical Microbiology

## T. J. J. Inglis

DM MRCPath DTM&H FRCPA
Medical Microbiologist, The Western Australian Centre for Pathology and
Medical Research, Nedlands, Western Australia

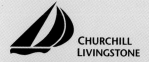

CHURCHILL
LIVINGSTONE

EDINBURGH LONDON MADRID MELBOURNE NEW YORK
SAN FRANCISCO AND TOKYO 1997

# Contents

# Preface

The information base required to practice medical microbiology has expanded considerably in the last decade. After more than a decade in microbiology my personal data stockpile includes one CD-ROM, around twenty major postgraduate textbooks, a large pile of specialist journals and an assortment of other sources, all of which are used regularly. The idea for this pocketbook grew out of discussions on how best to reduce the stockpile to a more manageable size.

My initial ideas were clarified and refined in discussions with Gamini Kumarasinghe, Kyle Webster and other colleagues in Singapore. The contents list began to gel during a brief appointment at the Norwich Public Health Laboratory, where Julia Roberts, Helen Williams, Phillipa White and Margaret Sillis gave me the benefit of their advice. Paul Hancock, Stephanie Stewart, and senior medical colleagues were largely responsible for keeping a more practical emphasis in view as the draft neared completion during the ensuing half year spent at Yeovil District Hospital. I am grateful to Mike Millar, a former sparring partner from Leeds, for his recommendations on the overall layout of contents. Thanks are also due to Annette MacFarlane, Patricia O'Neill and Rod Warren (Shrewsbury Public Health Laboratory) who worked with me on the infection control guidelines that appear in this book. The final draft was then read and checked by John Kurtz, Max Aravena-Roman and Moira Wilson after my move to PathCentre in Perth, W.A. Many other colleagues have contributed in one way or another at some stage of this project, not least in influencing the things I value most. I hope this pocketbook makes the help, kind advice and guidance from which I have benefitted more widely available.

This pocketbook should be kept close at hand in the laboratory, ward and clinic. It will be of greatest use if annotated with a record of new information you find helpful in the course of your work.

1997

T. J. J. I.

# Abbreviations

| | | | |
|---|---|---|---|
| ACDP | Advisory Committee on Dangerous Pathogens | EIA | enzyme immunoassay |
| ADH | arginine dehydrolase | EIEC | enteroinvaive *E. coli* |
| AFB | acid fast bacilli | EHEC | enterohaemorrhagic *E. coli* |
| APW | alkaline peptone water | ELISA | enzyme linked immunosorbent assay |
| AZT | azidothymidine | ENT | ear, nose and throat surgery |
| BAL | bronchoalveolar lavage | EORTC | European Oncology Research Trial Centre |
| BC | blood culture | EPEC | enteropathogenic *E. coli* |
| CAMP test | Augmented haemolysis specific to group B streptococci | ESR | erythrocyte sedimentation rate |
| CAPD | continuous ambulatory peritoneal dialysis | ETEC | enterotoxic *E. coli* |
| CCDC | Consultant in Communicable Disease Control | FDP | fibrin degradation products |
| CDC | Communicable Disease Centre | GMCSF | granulocyte macrophage colony stimulating factor |
| CFT | complement fixation text | GNB | Gram negative bacillus |
| CIN | cefsoludin irgasan novobiocin agar | GP | general practitioner |
| | | GPC | Gram positive coccus |
| CLED | cysteine lactose electrolyte deficient agar | HBV | hepatitis B virus |
| | | Hib | *Haemophilus influenzae* type B |
| CMV | cytomegalovirus | HIV | Human immunodeficiency virus |
| CSF | cerebrospinal fluid | | |
| CTS | cross sectional tomography scan | HMSO | Her Majesty's Stationery Office |
| CTA | cysteine tryptic digest agar | HSV | herpes simplex virus |
| | | HTLV | human T cell lymphotrophic virus |
| CXR | chest X-ray | IF | immunofluorescence |
| DGH | district general hospital | JEMBEC | James E Martin Biological Environmental Chamber |
| DGI | disseminated gonococcal infection | | |
| DIC | disseminated intravascular coagulation | KOH | potassium hydroxide |
| EBV | Epstein–Barr virus | LAP | leosine aminopeptidase |
| EEG | electroencephalogram | | |

| | | | |
|---|---|---|---|
| **LDC** | lysine decarboxylase | | tuberculosis |
| **LP** | lumbar puncture | **PYR** | pyrridonyl |
| **MAC** | MacConkey agar | | arylamidase |
| **MLSO** | Medical laboratory | **RBC** | red blood cell |
| | scientific officer | **RDT** | rapid diagnostic test |
| **MRI** | Magnetic resonance | **RF** | rheumatic fever |
| | imaging | **RIP** | rifampicin isoniazid |
| **MSU** | midstream specimen | | pyrazinamide |
| | of urine | **RSV** | respiratory syncytical |
| **NA** | nutrient agar | | virus |
| **NEQAS** | National External | **SMAC** | sorbitol MacConkey |
| | Quality Assurance | | agar |
| | Scheme | **STD** | sexually transmitted |
| **NP** | nosocomial | | disease |
| | pneumonia | **TCBS** | thiosulphate citrate |
| **ODC** | ornithine | | bile salt agar |
| | decarboxylase | **TSI** | triple sugar iron agar |
| **ONPG** | ortho-nitrophenyl | **UTI** | urinary tract infection |
| | galactose | **UV** | ultraviolet |
| **PCR** | polymerase chain | **VCNT** | vancomycin colistin |
| | reaction | | neomycin |
| **PPA** | phenylalanine | | trimethoprim agar |
| | deaminase | **VP** | Vosges–Proskauer test |
| **PPNG** | penicillinase | **WCC** | (total) White cell count |
| | producing *Neisseria* | **XLD** | xylose lysine |
| | *gonorrhoeae* | | decarboxylase agar |
| **PTB** | pulmonary | **ZN** | Zeihl–Neelsen stain |

# PROBLEM-BASED MICROBIOLOGY

# CENTRAL NERVOUS SYSTEM INFECTIONS

## ENCEPHALITIS, HSV

Definitive diagnosis of HSV encephalitis used to be by brain biopsy, with EEG or MRI to help localise the abnormal area. CSF, cytology and biochemistry are nonspecific. If available, PCR for HSV in CSF is now the preferred method. Culture from brain biopsy and treatment is usually started before confirmation of the diagnosis. Untreated, the mortality rate is up to 80% and a high proportion of survivors have major neurological sequelae.

### Treatment
Acyclovir 10 mg/kg i.v. every 8 hours for 2–3 weeks.

## MENINGITIS

Most meningitis deaths occur within two days of hospital admission, and have a bacterial aetiology.

---

**Aims**
- distinguish bacterial from viral infection
- recognise bacterial cause early.

**Need to know**
- patient's age
- details of any prior antibiotic therapy.

---

### Lumbar puncture contraindications
If there is evidence of raised intracranial pressure or intracranial mass, risk of uncal herniation following lumbar puncture (LP) dictates prior imaging studies (e.g. CT scan). Generalised infection and meningitis cause diffuse expansion and rarely result in herniation. Routine CT scan prior to LP can cause unnecessary delays in commencing emergency antibiotic therapy.

### CSF examination
Investigate as follows:

1. Macroscopic: is it turbid or bloodstained?
2. Add lytic stain to uncentrifuged aliquot.
3. Neutrophil/lymphocyte count in counting chamber.
4. Centrifuge further aliquot (2000 g × 10 min)..?xanthochromia.

5. Stain centrifuge deposit:
   - Gram (any bacteria are potentially significant)
   - Geimsa (% differential count)
   - Zeihl–Neelsen (if requested). NB around 25% sensitivity.
6. Inoculate deposit onto blood and chocolate agars, and in brain-heart infusion.
7. Antigen detection (latex, co-agglutination) if prior antibiotics or to confirm Gram stain result.

## CSF results (→ Table 1.1)

| TABLE 1.1 | Normal compared to abnormal CSF results | | | |
|---|---|---|---|---|
| Neutrophils/µl | Lymphocytes/µl | Protein(g/l) | Glucose/blood level | |
| 0 | ≤5 | <0.5 | 2/3 | Normal |
| >200–10 000 | <100 | >1 | <1/2 | Bacterial meningitis |
| <100 | 10–1000 | 0.5–1 | 2/3 | Viral meningitis |
| <100 | 50–1000 | 1–5 | <1/3 | Tuberculous meningitis |
| 5–100 | | >1 | 2/3 | Brain abscess |

## Difficulties and exceptions in CSF analysis

### CSF cell content

- No cells: some cases of early meningitis.
- Low neutrophil count but turbid CSF means a poor prognosis in pneumococcal meningitis.
- Lower neutrophil range in most cases of *Listeria* infection or raised lymphocytes instead (minority of cases).
- Artificially low count if CSF is collected in glass container.
- Other causes of raised count include: seizures, systemic viral infection, endocarditis.

### CSF chemistry

- Raised protein may be only indication of brain abscess.
- Glucose may fall in mumps (i.e. mumps meningitis), meningitis or lymphocytic choriomeningitis.

### Gram stain

- No bacteria in at least 10% cases, and 60% from community.
- Antigen detection may be no more sensitive than Gram stain.
- Scanty *H. influenzae* easily missed against fuchsin-stained proteinaceous background.

- *H. influenzae* may be confused with *S. pneumoniae* if poor decolourisation stage.
- *Listeria* can be confused with *S. pneumoniae* on initial stain.

## Therapeutic implications of CSF results

### 1. Presumptive therapy (→ Table 1.2)

**TABLE 1.2  Presumptive therapy in meningitis**

| Organism | Suggested presumptive therapy |
|---|---|
| Haemophilus influenzae | Ampicillin and chloramphenicol × 10 d (ampicillin 75 mg/kg i.v. + chloramphenicol 200 mg/kg i.m./i.v. per day) Alternative = cefotaxime 50 mg/kg per day |
| Neisseria meningitidis | Adult: benzyl penicillin × 5 d (2.4 g (4Mu) i.v. every 4 h) Child (1 month to 12 years): 180 –300 mg/kg daily total in 4–6 doses Alternative = chloramphenicol |
| Streptococcus pneumoniae | Benzyl penicillin × 14 d (2.4 g (2Mu) i.v. every 4 h) Alternative = cefotaxime, up to 300 mg/kg per day if penicillin resistant |
| Group B streptococcus | Benzyl penicillin and aminoglycoside i.v. (benzyl penicillin 150 mg/kg daily + gentamicin) |
| Escherichia coli | Ampicillin and aminoglycoside i.v. Alternative = ampicillin and cefotaxime |
| Listeria monocytogenes | Ampicillin and gentamicin i.v. |
| Cryptococcus neoformans | Amphoteracin B i.v. × 6 wk (amphoteracin 0.5–0.6 mg/kg daily +/– flucytosine 150 mg/kg daily) Alternative = fluconazole |
| Mycobacterium tuberculosis | Rifampicin, isoniazid, pyrazinamide po and streptomycin i.m. daily for 2–3 m, then drop streptomycin, continue others up to 1 yr |

### 2. Inconclusive CSF results but strong clinical suspicion
Commence therapy as follows:

- Neonate: ampicillin and gentamicin i.v.
- Infant to preschool child: ampicillin and chloramphenicol, or cefotaxime.
- Schoolchild to older adult: benzyl penicillin i.v., unless penicillin-resistant *S. pneumoniae* common.

### 3. Steroid therapy
Indications include:

- *H. influenzae* infection — give to reduce risk of neurological damage (deafness in circa 50%).
- *M. tuberculosis* — give to unconscious patients, infants with encephalitis and to halt spinal block.

### 4. Prophylaxis of close ('kissing') contacts

- Close *H. influenzae* and *N. meningitidis* contacts may benefit from rifampicin.
- *H. influenzae* contacts <4 years old — 10 mg/kg twice daily × 4 d.
- All close *N. meningitidis* contacts — 10 mg/kg (600 mg for adult) twice daily × 2 d. Alternative = cipofloxacin, single dose.

### Troubleshooting

Reasons for culture negative meningitis are:

- Viral infection.
- Antibiotic treatment started before LP.
- Mycobacterial infection.
- Cryptococcal infection.
- Intracranial abscess.

### Follow-up

Any positive or inconclusive CSF result justifies a follow-up visit, when preliminary culture results can be communicated directly to attending staff. This is a good opportunity to check:

- Was antibiotic therapy commenced?
- Was it appropriate?
- Has there been any clinical response?

## RABIES EXPOSURE

 **Although most cases arise from dog bites, other animals can transmit rabies.**

### Action

1. Scrub wound thoroughly with soap and water.
2. If bitten by domestic animal and owner available, arrange to have animal observed for 10 days.
3. If rabies transmission possible commence post-exposure prophylaxis:

### Previously unimmunised patient

Passive and active immunisation recommended.

- Active: human diploid cell vaccine (HDCV) 1.0 ml i.m. or s.c. into deltoid (anterolateral thigh in child). Repeat after 3, 7, 14, 30, 90 days.

- Passive: 20 iu/kg dose of rabies immunoglobulin, half infiltrated around the wound and half i.m.

*Previously immunised patient*

- HDCV 1.0 ml i.m. and repeat twice on days 0, 3–7.

4. Reassure patient that postexposure vaccination has a very high success rate even in a rabies outbreak.

# ENDOPHTHALMITIS

- A delay in treating endophthalmitis will increase the risk of permanent damage to the eye, and make eradication of infection more difficult.
- As Gram stain results can be misleading, presumptive therapy should be started on clinical grounds irrespective of microscopy.
- Vitreous humor is better than aqueous humor as a source of pathogens responsible for endophthalmitis, but the anterior chamber (and any stitch abscess or dehiscence) should still be sampled to increase the overall probability of a positive culture.
- Conjunctival cultures can be inaccurate and even misleading.

## Preparing to sample

You may be called to set up cultures and smears in the operating theatre. For this you will need:

- freshly cleaned (alcohol) microscope slides, and diamond
- blood, chocolate and Sabouraud's agar plates and marker pen
- sterile, disposable bacteriology loops
- slide box and plate rack
- request forms.

Also, if an automatic vitrectomy device is to be used, take some sterile syringes and bacterial filters, or take some sterile 20 ml plastic containers to bring back vitreous and aqueous specimens for filtration in the laboratory.

Culture has priority; if there is sufficient vitreous material, prepare smears for Gram stain, Geimsa, and periodic acid–Schiff (in that order).

## Unusual causes of endophthalmitis

- If fungal infection is suspected, ask the surgeon to sample any visible fluffballs and make sure you inoculate the Sabouraud's agar, and set up smears for either periodic acid – Schiff (PAS) or calcofluor white stains.
- If mycobacteria are suspected, examine a spun deposit of vitreous stained with auramine-phenol, and inoculate mycobacterial media.
- If toxoplasmosis is suspected, note cytology — often eosinophilic — and arrange serological investigations.

## Presumptive therapy (→ Table 1.3)

**TABLE 1.3  Presumptive therapy for endophthalmitis**

| Antibiotic | Intravitreal dose | Halflife inflamed | Uninflamed |
|---|---|---|---|
| Amikacin | 400 µg | ? | ? |
| Gentamicin | 200–400 µg | 40–60 h | 20–40 h |
| Vancomycin | 1000–2000 µg | 40–60 h | 48 h |
| Penicillin | 600 units | 8 | – |
| Ceftriaxone | 3000 µg | 15 h | 22 h |
| Clindamycin | 1000 µg | 6 h | – |
| Amphoteracin B | 5–10 µg in 0.1 ml | | |

The preferred presumptive regimen is intravitreal vancomycin plus an aminoglycoside (amikacin is said to be less retinotoxic than gentamicin), but most ophthalmologists still like to give systemic antibiotics as well. Additional subconjunctival antibiotics add little benefit.

### Follow-up
The initial Gram stain may not correspond to culture results; either:

- scanty bacteria visible on microscopy may refuse to grow
- a greater variety of bacterial species than anticipated may grow
- bacterial growth may follow an apparently clear Gram stain.

The conventional presumptive regimen may need repeating several times along with repeat vitrectomy to ensure sustained antibacterial activity.

# ENTERIC INFECTIONS

## General

The laboratory diagnosis of enteric infection is the microbiologist's equivalent of looking for a needle in a haystack; specimens come from the most heavily colonised site in the entire body, yet the possible pathogen must be separated out. The problem is compounded by the variety of enteric pathogens that may be encountered.

> **Remember**
> - The presence of a potential pathogen does not necessarily mean the presence of infection.
> - More than one enteric pathogen may be present.

## Specimen collection

Faeces should be passed into a dry, wide-mouthed container with a tight-fitting lid. Leakage in transit can put laboratory and other staff at risk of infection, and lead to deterioration of the specimen.

Patients are rarely instructed in how to collect the specimen. In hospital this can be done by recovering a sample from the bedpan, but patients at home should be warned against fishing material out of the lavatory pan. Plastic clingfilm can be placed as a loosely fitting cover over the lavatory. Alternatively, faeces can be passed into a clean/dry ice cream or margarine tub.

Contamination with urine, barium or bismuth should be avoided. At least one week should have passed between barium enema and stool collection for enteric parasites. Prolonged transport time can lead to the reduced viability of some pathogens (e.g. *Shigella* spp.) because faecal pH falls with temperature. Specimens for diagnosis of amoebic dysentery must be examined while still warm if motile trophozoites are to be seen.

The string test may be used to obtain duodenal material for diagnosis of giardiasis or strongyloidiasis. Bile staining of the string is an indication that a satisfactory length has been swallowed.

## Specimen processing

### Mandatory tests

These include:

- microscopy for cryptosporidiosis
- direct faecal smear for enteric parasites
- culture for *Salmonella, Shigella* and *Campylobacter* spp. [suggested media: XLD + Hektoen + Skirrow's].

*Optional tests (→ Table 1.4)*

**TABLE 1.4   Optional tests for enteric infections**

| Indication | Test | Media |
|---|---|---|
| Diarrhoea, infant or travel | E. coli culture | MAC |
| Bloody diarrhoea | E.coli 0157 | SMAC |
| Diarrhoea, overseas travel | Vibrio culture | TCBS, APW |
| Salmonella carrier, food handler | Salmonella enrichment | Selenite broth |
| Mesenteric adenitis | Yersinia culture | CIN |
| Diarrhoea, child, seasonal | Rotavirus ELISA | |
| Diarrhoea, overseas travel, immunocompromised | Mircroscopy, faeces concentrate | |
| Diarrhoea, antibiotics | C. difficile toxin | |

 No single agar medium is ideal for screening of faeces for the more common bacterial pathogens. Most laboratories use two for *Salmonella* and *Shigella*, and a third for *Campylobacter* spp.)

Other media should be added at the put-up stage according to clinical information supplied on the request form.

Many cases of viral enteritis are due to rotavirus, which can be rapidly diagnosed by antigen detection ELISA. The latex agglutination test is specific but far less sensitive. If available, tests for other viral enteric pathogens should be performed, when rotavirus is negative.

## Microscopic appearance of intestinal parasites

Commonly encountered intestinal parasites are recognised on microscopy and depicted in Figure 1.1. Other intestinal parasites including protozoa and shistosome eggs are depicted in Figure 1.2. Features used to differentiate hookworm and strongyloides larvae are shown in Figure 1.3.

## Presumptive identification of bacterial pathogens

### XLD

- Black colonies may be *Salmonella*. Do urease to exclude *Proteus* sp. and oxidase to exclude *Pseudomonas*. If both are negative do biochemical tests to confirm.
- Pink colonies may be *Salmonella* or *Shigella*. Do urease to exclude *Proteus* sp. then biochemical tests to confirm.
- Yellow colonies, if oxidase positive, may be *Aeromonas*. Biochemical tests required to confirm.

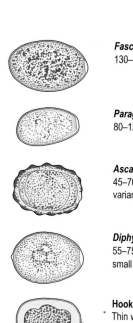

**Fasciola hepatica**
130–150 µm, inconspicuous operculum

**Paragonimus westermanii**
80–120 µm, slightly shouldered operculum

**Ascaris lumbricoides (fertile)**
45–70 µm, marmillated thick outer wall; infertile
variant more elongated: 85–95 mm

**Diphylobothrium latum**
55–75 µm, inconspicuous operculum,
small knob at opposite end

**Hookworm**
Thin walled ovum, 55–75 µm,
usually partly embryonated

**Enterobius vermicularis**
50–60 µm, asymetrical, thick walled ovum

**Trichuris trichuria**
50–55 µm, thick walled, lemon-shaped
plugs at both ends

**Tinea spp.**
30–45 µm, striated outer layer

**Clonorchis sinensis**
25–35 µm, shouldered operculum

**Fig. 1.1** Commonly encountered intestinal parasites.

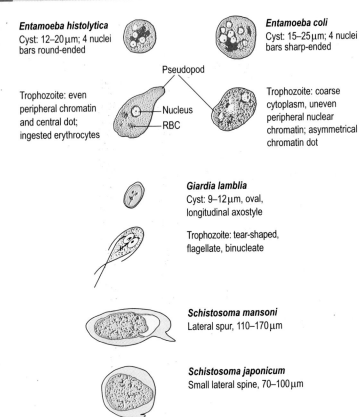

**Entamoeba histolytica**
Cyst: 12–20 μm; 4 nuclei
bars round-ended

**Entamoeba coli**
Cyst: 15–25 μm; 4 nuclei
bars sharp-ended

Trophozoite: even
peripheral chromatin
and central dot;
ingested erythrocytes

Pseudopod

Nucleus

RBC

Trophozoite: coarse
cytoplasm, uneven
peripheral nuclear
chromatin; asymmetrical
chromatin dot

**Giardia lamblia**
Cyst: 9–12 μm, oval,
longitudinal axostyle

Trophozoite: tear-shaped,
flagellate, binucleate

**Schistosoma mansoni**
Lateral spur, 110–170 μm

**Schistosoma japonicum**
Small lateral spine, 70–100 μm

**Fig. 1.2** Intestinal protozoa and shistosome eggs.

*Hektoen enteric* The basic algorithm is the same as for XLD except pink on XLD equals green on Hektoen.

*Agglutination tests* These should not be performed on colonies picked directly from selective media. Instead they should be subcultured onto nonselective media e.g. blood agar.

● Smaller laboratories will only test Salmonella polyvalent O, poly H and Vi, and report '*Salmonella* sp' (Table 1.5).
● Larger laboratories may carry a fuller set of antisera, e.g. RDT, and more common specific O and H. Polyvalent antisera to the 4 species of Shigella are usually sufficient (Table 1.6).

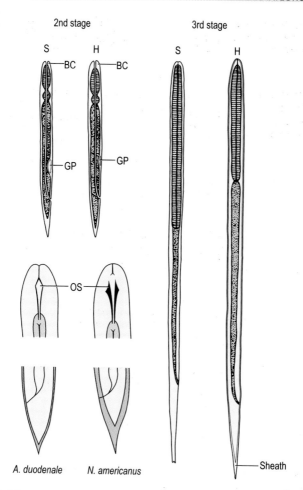

**Fig. 1.3** Differentiation between hookworm and strongyloides larvae. (S, strongyloides; H, hookworm; BC, buccal capsule; GP, genital primordium; OS, oesophageal spears.) (Redrawn with permission from Zaman V, Keong L 1989 *Handbook of medical parasitology* Churchill Livingstone, Edinburgh)

*Campylobacter media* After incubation under microaerophilic conditions at 41°C, oxidase positive colonies are usually *Campylobacter* sp. Confirmation may require incubation on blood agar at 41°C both aerobically and

**TABLE 1.5    Agglutination reactions of Salmonellas**

| Serotype | Reactions | |
|---|---|---|
| S. enteritidis | O 1,9,12: | H g,m:- |
| S. typhimurium | O 1,4,5,12: | H i:1,2 |
| S. virchow | O 6,7: | H r: 1,2 |
| S. hadar | O 6,8: | H $z_{10}$:e,n,x |
| S. indiana | O 1,4,12: | H z: 1,7 |
| S. newport | O 6,8: | H e, h: 1,2 |
| S. infantis | O 6,7[14]: | H r: 1,5 |
| S. heidelberg | O [1] 4[5]12: | H r: 1,2 |
| S. poona | O [1]13,22[37] | H z: 1,6 |
| S. braenderup | O 6,7 | H e, h: e,n,$z_{15}$ |
| **Enteric fever salmonellas** | | |
| S. typhi | O 9,12[Vi] | H d:- |
| S. paratyphi A | O 1,2,12: | H a:- |
| S. paratyphi B | O 1,4,5,12: | H b: 1,2 |
| S. paratyphi C | O 6,7[Vi]: | H c: 1,5 |
| S. choleraesuis | O 6,7: | H c: 1,5 |

**TABLE 1.6    Shigella spp. agglutinating antisera**

First line
- S. dysenteriae polyvalent 1–10.
- S. flexner polyvalent.
- S. boydii polyvalent 1–15.
- S. sonnei phase 1, 2.

Second line
- Specific antisera for more common serotypes of all Shigella spp. apart from S. sonnei
- S. flexner has a complex system that requires a large number of antisera types for subtyping

microaerophilically, with an erythromycin disk on the plate. Species level identification is not usually required.

### E. coli Lactose fermenter on MAC.

- Enterotoxic strains can be confirmed by heat stable and labile toxin assay in reference labs.
- Enteropathogenic strains should be sought by using O55 and O111 antisera only during outbreaks in neonatal units.
- Enterohaemorrhagic strains can be sought by culture on sorbitol MAC; they are nonfermenters, and β-glucuronidase/MUG negative.

*Vibrio cholerae* Yellow colonies on thiosulphate-citrate bile salt-sucrose. Subculture to nonselective agar before performing oxidase: positive, GNB, with positive string test (*Aeromonas* sp. is string test negative) agglutinating antisera and biochemical tests are needed for confirmation.

> Subculture to alkaline peptone water, after 6 h incubation at 37°C from top of unstirred APW onto TCBS; oxidase reaction off TCBS may produce false negative.

*Vibrio parahaemolyticus* Green colonies on TCBS, oxidase positive GNB. Confirmation by biochemical reactions.

*Clostridium difficile* Culture though possible is not considered helpful in diagnosis of antibiotic associated colitis due to high level of faecal carriage.

*Helicobacter pylori* Small colonies appear after several days on blood agar in microaerophilic conditions at 37°C; oxidase and catalase positive, and rapid urease positive.

*Yersinia sp.* Growth on CIN agar produces pink-centred colonies after 48 h with translucent edges. Biochemical confirmation is required, if on MAC. Small colonies appear after 24 h, that enlarge at room temperature.

## Campylobacters

Most clinical isolates of diarrhoea-associated *Campylobacter* sp. from selective campylobacter medium incubated microaerophilically will be *C. jejuni* subsp. *jejuni*. Unless further tests are performed, refer to these as '*Campylobacter* sp.'.

> - Conditions used to detect campylobacters in faeces will miss many *C. foetus* subsp. *foetus* and *C. upsaliensis*.
> - Human disease is occasionally caused by *C. lari* and *C. hyointestinalis* both of which are nalidixic acid sensitive.

## Vibrios

Most epidemic cholera is caused by O:1 *Vibrio cholerae*. Non-O:1 *V. cholerae* (group 2–6) may cause cholera but not in outbreaks. Separation of *V. cholerae* into Classical and El Tor biotypes, and into Ogawa, Inaba and Hikojima serotypes should be performed by reference labs with an epidemiological interest in vibrio diseases.

Presumptive confirmation of *V. cholerae* can be done with a combination of TCBS agar, oxidase from subculture on nonselective agar, sensitivity to the vibriostatic agent 0/129, and specific agglutination reaction. Identification of other *Vibrio* spp. may be performed with commercial biochemical identification kits but suspensions of the test organism must be made up in 0.89% NaCl.

 **V. metchnikoffii is oxidase negative.**

### Indications for antibiotic therapy in patients with diarrhoea

1. Enteric fever, *S. typhi/paratyphi* isolated. [NB Aminoglycosides and cephalosporins have poor clinical effect despite appearing sensitive under lab conditions.]
2. Bacillary or amoebic dysentery.
3. Haemorrhagic colitis, during the acute infective stage.
4. Severe diarrhoea at both extremes of age.
5. Cholera. Antibiotics may reduce severity and duration.
6. Parasitic infections such as giardiasis, amoebiasis and strongyloidiasis.
7. Salmonella carriage in food handlers.

However, most instances of salmonella, *S. sonnei* and campylobacter infection do not require antibiotic treatment.

### Management of inpatients with viral enteritis

- Fluid and electrolyte replacement is vital and with good nursing support can be achieved using oral rehydration solution (ORS) in many cases.
- Feeding should be started within 24 h to promote intestinal epithelial regeneration.
- Patients should be nursed in a single-bed sideward with enteric precautions and sent home as soon as possible.
- If an outbreak occurs on a ward, it should be closed to further admissions.

### Follow-up

There are three main requirements in the follow-up of enteric infection:

- making sure patients who need antibiotic treatment are given the appropriate agents
- making sure those who do not need treatment do not get given antibiotics unnecessarily
- making sure that there is no secondary spread of enteric infection.

Any patient with a specific enteric infection while in hospital warrants a visit by the medical microbiologist for the above reasons. Infection control precautions may not have been instituted, and the infection control team may be unaware of the problem.

Patients with enteric infections in general practice usually do not require antibiotic treatment, but the appropriate GP and the CCDC should both be informed because of public health implications.

## Infection control precautions

These are mainly for:

- infectious diarrhoea
- 'gastroenteritis'
- salmonellosis, shigellosis, cryptosporidiosis
- rotavirus and other viral enteric infections
- enteric fever (typhoid/paratyphoid)
- cholera.

Under standard and additional precautions (see below) standard measures are adequate for enteric infections, but for patients who are younger than 6 years, incontinent or in nappies, contact precautions will also be required.

### Protocol

1. A high standard of hand hygiene should be observed by all staff working on or visiting the unit.
2. Plain soap may be a better handwash agent than chlorhexidine for some (viral) enteric pathogens.
3. Consumption of food, smoking and application of makeup should be avoided by staff in or near the affected unit.
4. Faeces and vomit should be disposed of as infected waste — i.e. handled by staff with gloved hands and wearing disposable plastic aprons — and covered with a phenolic disinfectant before disposal in the sluice.
5. Spills of infected material should be soaked with a phenolic disinfectant, left for 30 min covered with paper towels, and then wiped up.
6. Bedding should be treated as infected and decontaminated by a hot wash cycle. It may be more convenient to discard heavily soiled bedding as infected waste.
7. A single-bed sideward is only mandatory if the patient is incontinent of faeces, or has dangerously poor personal hygiene.

 **A locally agreed protocol may be available in the nursing procedures book on the ward.**

# FEVER

## INITIAL WORKUP

> **Aims:**
> - Search for a specific aetiological diagnosis that will help guide therapeutic decision-making.
> - Make progress with essential diagnostic tests without delaying presumptive therapy.
>
> **Remember:** you cannot get every relevant test done on call.

The middle of the night is not the best time to begin an investigation into the cause of a febrile episode. A public holiday or weekend is even worse. Investigations should be limited to what can be performed on call and advice restricted to easily remembered **key points**.

Avoid dictating detailed management protocols out of hours. It is better to call again later or make a **follow-up visit** to the ward, when the passage of time, a wider repertoire of investigations and daylight can all illuminate the clinical problem in question.

Calls will only rarely be made to request a **diagnostic opinion** out of hours. When they are, it will usually be to sort out a problem the attending physician/surgeon is either unwilling or unable to resolve. You should therefore enquire about what is known/has been done already, without criticising your clinical colleagues or promising an immediate solution.

More often, the clinical problem will be drawn to your attention as a **side issue** while you answer a call about an urgent specimen (e.g. blood culture or CSF) or help with the interpretation of a test result (e.g. out-of-range aminoglycoside level). You may therefore only have time to ask the one or two most relevant questions from the following list:

### History

- Age (paediatric or geriatric).
- Main reason for hospital admission.
- Date of admission (?nosocomial infection).
- Overseas travel, human contact or animal handling.
- Prior/intended antibiotic therapy.

### Examination

- Temperature.
- Any localising features.

## Investigations

- Total/differential white cell count.
- ESR or C-reactive protein.
- Chest X-ray/other diagnostic imaging.
- Recent microbiology tests.

## Specimen priority

There are few truly rapid microbiological tests that have an immediate impact on therapeutic decision-making. Most of these are either microscopy or antigen detection. Bacteriological cultures must be started before commencing empirical therapy if at all possible, though results may take a day or so to come through. Serological investigations should not be significantly affected by antibiotic therapy or a 12-hour delay. They can usually wait until the laboratory reopens.

## NEUTROPOENIC PATIENTS

The risk of bacterial and yeast infection rises with the severity of neutropoenia and is particularly high when neutrophil count falls below $5 \times 10^5$/ml.

The skin and gastrointestinal tract are thought to be the most common source of infection. Presumptive antibiotic therapy should therefore be directed against organisms from these sites.

EORTC multicentre studies have highlighted the need for initial intravenous, broad spectrum antibiotics. Many centres use a combination of aminoglycoside and β-lactam agents, e.g. gentamicin and piperacillin.

Where skin or intravascular cannula infections are suspected as a cause of fever, antibiotics effective against coagulase negative staphylococci should be used, e.g. vancomycin, unless there are antibiotic sensitivities. Some centres use vancomycin as part of the initial presumptive therapy, but this should be discouraged where possible due to the risk of selecting vancomycin resistant enterococci, which may subsequently cause untreatable infections.

If the patient has not responded to antibacterial agents within 48 hours, the need for antifungal therapy should be considered.

Some patients may not respond to optimal antibiotic therapy until their neutrophil count begins to rise again. Occasionally, it may be necessary to use GMCSF to obtain a favourable response to anti-infective therapy.

## RETURNING TRAVELLERS

## ARBOVIRUS INFECTION

Endemic areas include:

- Chikungunya fever: Africa, parts of Southeast Asia.

- Congo-Crimean haemorrhagic fever: Eastern Europe, Middle East, Asia, all Africa.
- Dengue, DHF: tropical and subtropical Africa, Asia, Australia, Americas including urban centres where *Aedes aegypti* mosquito is present.
- Ebola fever: outbreaks in Kenya, Zaire, Sudan.
- Epidemic polyarthritis (Ross river virus): North and Eastern Australia, Irian Jaya, Papua New Guinea, islands in Western Pacific.
- Group C virus fevers: Brazil, other parts of South America.
- Japanese encephalitis: widespread in rural South and East Asia.
- Kyasanur forest disease: northern India.
- Lassa fever: West Africa.
- Marburg haemorrhagic fever: few cases in Kenya, Zimbabwe, RSA.
- Mayaro fever: Trinidad, Surinam, Brazil, Bolivia.
- O'nyong nyong fever: tropical Africa.
- Oropouche fever: Brazil.
- Rift valley fever: sub-Saharan Africa.
- Rochio encephalitis: Brazil.
- Sandfly (papatasi) fever: Mediterranean littoral.
- Sindbis fever: sporadic outbreaks in Uganda, South Africa, Scandinavia, Russia, Australia.
- Venezuelan equine encephalitis: northern parts of South America, Central America.
- Yellow fever: tropical South America and Africa (*not present* in Asia, the pacific islands or Australia).

## MALARIA

Malaria risk (→ Table 1.7)

**TABLE 1.7   Areas of malaria risk**

| Country | Malaria risk | Resistance |
|---|---|---|
| **North Africa/Middle East** | | |
| Abu Dhabi | Very low | |
| Afghanistan | Present | Chloroquine |
| Algeria | Very low | |
| Azerbaijan | Low | |
| Egypt (most) | Very low | |
| Egypt (El Faiyum) | Low | |
| Iran | Present | Chloroquine |
| Iraq (north) | Low | |
| Libya | Very low | |
| Morocco | Very low | |
| Oman | Present | Chloroquine |
| Saudi Arabia | Present | Chloroquine |

**TABLE 1.7    Areas of malaria risk (cont'd)**

| | | |
|---|---|---|
| Syria (north) | Low | |
| Tajikistan (south) | Low | |
| Tunisia | Very low | |
| Turkey (most) | Very low | |
| Turkey (Adona, Side, SE Anatolia) | Low | |
| U.A.E. | Present | Chloroquine |
| Yemen | Present | Chloroquine |
| **Sub-Saharan Africa** | | |
| Angola | High | Chloroquine widespread |
| Benin | High | Chloroquine widespread |
| Botswana | Present in parts | Chloroquine |
| Burkina Fasso | High | Chloroquine widespread |
| Burundi | High | Chloroquine widespread |
| Cameroon | High | Chloroquine widespread |
| C.A.R. | High | Chloroquine widespread |
| Cape Verde | Low | |
| Chad | High | Chloroquine widespread |
| Comoros | High | Chloroquine widespread |
| Congo | High | Chloroquine widespread |
| Djibouti | High | Chloroquine widespread |
| Eritrea | High | Chloroquine widespread |
| Equ. Guinea | High | Chloroquine widespread |
| Ethiopia | High | Chloroquine widespread |
| Gabon | High | Chloroquine widespread |
| Gambia | High | Chloroquine widespread |
| Guinea | High | Chloroquine widespread |
| Guinea-Bissau | High | Chloroquine widespread |
| Ivory Coast | High | Chloroquine widespread |
| Kenya | High | Chloroquine widespread |
| Liberia | High | Chloroquine widespread |
| Madagascar | High | Chloroquine widespread |
| Malawi | High | Chloroquine widespread |
| Mali | High | Chloroquine widespread |
| Mauritania | Present in parts | Chloroquine |
| Mauritius | Low | |
| Mozambique | High | Chloroquine widespread |
| Namibia | Present in parts | Chloroquine |
| Niger | High | Chloroquine widespread |
| Nigeria | High | Chloroquine widespread |
| Principe | High | Chloroquine widespread |

**TABLE 1.7  Areas of malaria risk (cont'd)**

| | | |
|---|---|---|
| Rwanda | High | Chloroquine widespread |
| Sao Tome | High | Chloroquine widespread |
| Senegal | High | Chloroquine widespread |
| Sierra Leone | High | Chloroquine widespread |
| Somalia | High | Chloroquine widespread |
| South Africa | Present in parts | Chloroquine |
| Sudan | High | Chloroquine widespread |
| Swaziland | High | Chloroquine widespread |
| Tanzania | High | Chloroquine widespread |
| Togo | High | Chloroquine widespread |
| Uganda | High | Chloroquine widespread |
| Zaire | High | Chloroquine widespread |
| Zambia | High | Chloroquine widespread |
| Zimbabwe | Present in parts | Chloroquine |
| **South Asia** | | |
| Bangladesh (east) | High | Chloroquine |
| Bangladesh | Variable | Chloroquine |
| Bhutan (southern) | Variable | Chloroquine |
| India | Variable | Chloroquine |
| Nepal | Variable | Chloroquine |
| Pakistan | Variable | Chloroquine |
| Sri Lanka | Variable | Chloroquine |
| **Southeast Asia** | | |
| Burma | Substantial | Chloroquine |
| Cambodia | Substantial | Chloroquine |
| Cambodia, western | High | Chloroquine, mefloquine |
| China | Very low | |
| China (Yunnan, Hainan) | Substantial | Chloroquine |
| Hong Kong | Very low | |
| Indonesia | | |
| Bali | Very low | |
| Java | Variable | Chloroquine |
| Sumatra | Variable | Chloroquine |
| Irian Jaya | Substantial | Chloroquine |
| Laos | Substantial | Chloroquine |
| Malaysia, peninsula | Very low | |
| Sabah | Substantial | Chloroquine |
| Sarawak | Variable | Chloroquine |
| Philippines | Variable | Chloroquine |
| Thailand, main resorts | Very low | |
| Thailand, rural | Substantial | Chloroquine |
| Thailand, N borders | High | Chloroquine, mefloquine |
| Vietnam | Substantial | Chloroquine |

| TABLE 1.7 Areas of malaria risk (cont'd) | | |
| --- | --- | --- |
| **Oceania** | | |
| Papua New Guinea | High | Chloroquine |
| Solomon Islands | High | Chloroquine |
| Vanuatu | High | Chloroquine |
| **Central and South America** | | |
| Argentina | Variable | |
| Belize | Variable | |
| Bolivia | Variable | Chloroquine |
| Brazil (Amazon basin) | High | Chloroquine |
| Colombia | High | Chloroquine |
| Costa Rica | Variable | |
| Dominican Republic | Variable | |
| Ecuador | Variable | Chloroquine |
| El Salvador | Variable | |
| French Guiana | High | Chloroquine |
| Guatemala | Variable | |
| Guyana | High | Chloroquine |
| Haiti | Variable | |
| Honduras | Variable | |
| Mexico | Variable | |
| Nicaragua | Variable | |
| Panama | Variable | Chloroquine |
| Paraguay | Variable | |
| Peru | Variable | Chloroquine |
| Surinam | High | Chloroquine |
| Venezuela | Variable | Chloroquine |

[Malaria risk data quoted from: Bradley DJ, Warhurst DC 1995 Malaria prophylaxis: guidelines for travellers from Britain. BMJ 310: 709–714]

## Laboratory confirmation

Blood smears for malaria should be prepared beside the patient if possible. If malaria is suspected, at least two thin films should be made during a 24-hour period especially if fever has become intermittent. Patients with suspected chronic malaria, partially treated disease or other reason for low level parasitaemia should also have a thick film prepared. Thick films are much more sensitive than thin films, but require an experienced microscopist to interpret them. Filariasis may require a smear prepared late at night to coincide with the peak parasitaemia.

Key questions are:
- Has the patient got malaria?
- Is malaria due to *Plasmodium falciparum*?

The majority of fatal malaria infections are due to *Plasmodium falciparum*. As malignant falciparum malaria has a short incubation period and is not associated with prolonged chronic disease or relapse after a disease-free interval, a careful travel history including exposure to biting insects will help assess the likelihood of exposure to *P. falciparum*.

Two blood films should be collected, as discussed above, but if there is any doubt, repeat films are indicated. Thick films are more sensitive, but interpretation difficulties make the thin film, if positive, more suitable for differentiating *Plasmodium* spp. on their morphological features (see Fig. 1.4).

## Morphological pointers in the four species (Fig. 1.4)

### 1. *Pl. falciparum*

- High proportion of red cells with trophozoites.
- Accolé form trophozoites.
- Small, double nuclei trophozoites.
- Multiple trophozoites per red blood cell.
- Gametocytes rarely present in acute disease.
- Banana-shaped male gametocyte.
- Schizonts very rarely present.

### 2. *Pl. vivax*

- Ring form, early trophozoites usually single/RBC.
- Double chromatin dot rare.
- Schuffner's dots.
- Infected red blood cells enlarged.
- Amoeboid later trophozoites.
- Schizonts (multiple nuclei) and gametocytes visible in established infection.)

**Fig. 1.4** Morphological features of *Plasmodium* spp.

*P. falciparum.* 1) Early trophozoite (Accole form). 2) Early trophozoite double infection. 3) Early trophozoite double chromatin with a few Maurer's dots. 4) Late trophozoite with Maurer's dots and crenated red cell. 5) Mature schizont with merozoites and clumped pigment. 6) Macrogametocyte with bluish cytoplasm and compact chromatin. 7) Microgametocyte with pinkish cytoplasm and dispersed chromatin.

*P. vivax.* 1) Early trophozoite (ring form) with Schuffner's dots. 2) Late trophozoite with Schuffner's dots and enlarged red cell. 3) Late trophozoite with amoeboid cytoplasm. 4) Late trophozoite with amoeboid cytoplasm. 5) Mature schizont with merozoites and clumped pigment. 6) Microgametocyte with irregular nucleus. 7) Macrogametocyte with compact nucleus.

*P. malariae.* 1) Early trophozoite (ring form). 2) Early trophozoite with central chromatin. 3) Early trophozoite form. 4) Late trophozoite band form with distinct pigment. 5) Mature schizont with merozoite forming a rosette. 6) Microgametocyte with irregular nucleus. 7) Macrogametocyte with compact nucleus.

*P. ovale.* 1) Early trophozoite (ring form) with Schuffner's dots. 2) Developing schizont with enlarged red cell and Schuffner's dots. 3) Developing schizont in a red cell with jagged edges. 4) Developing schizont in an irregular red cell. 5) Mature schizont with merozoites arranged irregularly. 6) Microgametocyte with irregular nucleus. 7) Macrogametocyte with compact nucleus. (Reproduced with permission from Zaman V, Keong L 1989 *Handbook of medical parasitology* Churchill Livingstone, Edinburgh)

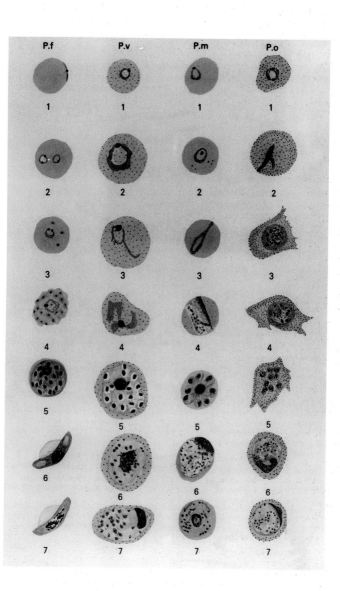

3. *Pl. malariae*

- Early trophozoites are small ring forms.
- Mature trophozoites are band forms.
- Infected red cells not enlarged, no Schuffner's dots.
- Small schizonts, max 10 merozoites, central malaria pigment.
- Gametocytes similar to *Pl. vivax*

4. Pl. ovale (mainly W. Africa)

- Infected red cells enlarged, sometimes oval, irregular edge.
- Schuffner's dots usually present with older trophozoites.
- Schizonts; max 8 merozoites inside, central malaria pigment.

## Malaria treatment guidelines (→ Table 1.8)

Chemotherapy of severe falciparum malaria involves parenteral quinidine or quinine in one of the following four regimes:

1. Quinidine (base) 6.2 mg/kg loading dose (quinidine gluconate [salt] 10 mg/kg) by intravenous infusion over 1–2 h, followed by quinidine (base) 0.0125 mg/kg/min (quinidine gluconate [salt] 0.02 mg/kg per min) by infusion pump.
2. Quinidine (base) 15 mg/kg loading dose (quinidine gluconate [salt] 24 mg/kg) by intravenous infusion over 4 h, followed by quinidine (base) 7.5 mg/kg (quinidine gluconate [salt] 12 mg/kg) every 8 h infused over 4 h.
3. Quinine (base) 16.7 mg/kg loading dose (quinine dihydrochloride [salt] 20 mg/kg) by intravenous infusion over 4 h, followed by quinine (base) 8.3 mg/kg (quinine dihydrochloride [salt] 10 mg/kg) every 8 h infused over 4 h.
4. Quinine (base) 5.8 mg/kg loading dose (quinine dihydrochloride [salt] 7 mg/kg) intravenously by infusion pump over 30 min, followed immediately by quinine (base) 8.3 mg/kg (quinine dihydrochloride [salt] 10 mg/kg) infused over 4 h, repeated 8-hourly.

From Kain CK, Gadd E, Gushulak B, MacCarthy A, MacPherson D, on behalf of the Committee to Advise on Tropical Health and Travel (CATMAT), Health and Welfare, Canada. 1996 Errors in treatment recommendations for severe malaria. Lancet 348: 621

---

**TABLE 1.8    Notes on malarial treatment**

- Oral quinine should be substituted as soon as possible. In patients requiring more than 48 h parenteral therapy, reduce the maintenance dose by one-third to one-half
- Loading dose must be omitted in patients who have received quinine, quinidine or mefloquine in the preceding 24 hours
- A second active agent such as doxycycline or Fansidar is added to complete therapy
- With quinidine therapy, electrocardiographic monitoring is necessary to detect cardiac arrhythmias

## Malaria prophylaxis

> **Remember:**
> - Prophylaxis is less than 100% effective against infection with *Plasmodium* spp. Personal protection measures are the most important aspect of prevention.
> - Prophylaxis should be started 1–2 weeks before departure, and continued for at least 4 weeks following return.

For short-term exposure 300 mg chloroquine (base) weekly is commonly used. This may be satisfactory where no resistance has been reported and the overall malaria risk is low. However, a higher risk may justify halving the tablets and taking them daily to ensure a more reliable shizontocidal effect.

Where chloroquine resistance is present but uncommon, 200 mg proguanil HCl is recommended as well as chloroquine. Both can be taken in pregnancy, but folate supplements should also be taken. Proguanil has an additive causal (pre-erythrocytic) prophylactic effect greater than in vitro tests might suggest.

If there is a significant risk of chloroquine resistance, the prophylactic agent of choice is mefloquine 250 mg weekly. An alternative should be used if there is a history of epilepsy or other major neuro/psychiatric illness. Proguanil and doxycycline have been used for this purpose in some settings.

Should malaria prophylaxis be required for more than one year, for travel in areas where the risk of exposure is great, or during the first trimester of pregnancy, it is wise to seek specialist advice.

Malaria prophylaxis is a complex issue, particularly as new and established forms of resistance are becoming common at the same time as travel to exotic tropical destinations becomes more popular.
**Remember:**
- Chemoprophylaxis does not provide 100% protection.
- Travellers still need to avoid mosquito bites.
- Travellers should continue taking their tablets for 4 weeks after returning.
- Malaria may still occur several months after returning.

## VIRAL HAEMORRHAGIC FEVER

Human-to-human transmission of Lassa, Ebola and Marburg agents is unknown outside Africa. Nevertheless, these are all biohazard level 4 viral pathogens and require the highest level of biocontainment.

## Procedure

Patients should not be admitted until assessed by CCDC or a consultant specialising in tropical medicine. If admitted before assessment, they should be kept in a single room and other staff prevented from entering until the patient has been seen by the above specialist. If admitted via the accident and emergency department, the patient should be put in a single room equipped with a box of protective clothing.

### Important differential diagnoses

Consider severe malaria and typhoid fever.

### Grading

The probability of viral haemorrhagic fever should be graded as strong, moderate or minimal (→ Table 1.9). It is very unlikely that a patient from a major city will have viral haemorrhagic fever.

| TABLE 1.9 | Levels of security for haemorrhagic fever |
| --- | --- |
| Grade | Containment |
| Strong: | High security isolation unit |
| | Surveillance of contacts |
| Moderate: | Regional infectious disease unit |
| Minimal: | Regional unit, or DGH isolation unit |

Laboratory specimens should all be handled in a biohazard level 4 lab, with the exception of a blood film for malaria, which should first be decontaminated with formalin. Urine and faeces should be discarded as high risk contaminated waste and either treated with hypochlorite before incineration, or autoclaved. Patients must be transferred between units in a specially equipped ambulance.

# GENITAL INFECTIONS

- More than one sexually transmitted infection may be present.
- Specimen quality and duration of transport have a direct bearing on the likelihood of laboratory confirmation of infection.

## Specimen collection

### Male urethra

Express excess exudate from urethra, clean with swab and discard, then insert fine dacron or alginate swab 2–3 cm into urethra and leave for a few seconds to absorb exudate. Next, insert further swab for chlamydias, rotate one full turn and withdraw. If no discharge at all, get patient to return for early morning specimen after 12 h water fast and before passing urine.

If symptoms suggest prostatitis, clean glans with soap and water, massage prostate via rectum and either collect urine specimens before and after massage, or swab exudate.

### Cervix

The uterine cervix should be examined using an unlubricated speculum if at all possible. Then use a large cotton swab to remove excess exudate and cervical mucus. Discard the cleaning swab. Insert the sampling swab a few millimetres past the os cervix. A further swab is required for chlamydias. This should come into vigorous contact with the endocervical columnar epithelium. Neither swab should be allowed to brush against the vaginal wall or touch the speculum. Swabs should also be collected from the urethra and rectum in all female patients suspected of gonococcal or chlamydial disease.

### Female urethra

Remove exudate from orifice with a cleaning swab. Use a sampling swab to collect discharge after massaging urethra against the symphysis pubis. If there is no exudate, wash the urethral orifice thoroughly and insert a fine urethral swab.

### Vagina

Vaginal exudate should be sampled from the posterior fornix with the aid of a speculum, after removing excess with a cleaning swab. The consistency and smell may give some indication of an infective aetiology:

- Frothy/offensive — *Trichomonas vaginalis*
- Thick and cheesy — *Candida albicans*
- Thin/slightly fishy — bacterial vaginosis.

*Genital ulcer exudate*

Touch a glass microscope slide against the ulcer base for immediate microscopy. A duplicate will be useful. If the ulcers are multiple, small and sometimes vesicular (i.e. genital herpes is a possible diagnosis), clean the ulcer surface with sterile cotton swab and sample the base of the ulcer with a virology swab. Alternatively, if vesicles are present, use a small syringe and fine needle to aspirate vesicle fluid for viral culture.

## Immediate specimen handling and transport

Where possible, transport and culture media should be inoculated immediately after specimen collection, and at the same time as smear preparations are made for subsequent microscopy. Genitourinary medicine clinics should be supplied with specimen collection packs containing all the swabs, microscope slides, transport media and agar plates required. JEMBEC or Transgrow packs that allow transport of inoculated agar plates in a $CO_2$-rich atmosphere increase the yield of positive gonococcal cultures. Specific transport media are required for chlamydias and for virus culture.

- Chlamydias should be kept cool, and in transit for only a short period.
- Herpes simplex virus is very prone to drying.
- If transport media is to be used for mycoplasma/ureaplasma culture, do not break the swab (plasticisers may be inhibitory) but inoculate medium by agitating the swab instead.

Prolonged transport times for genital exudate specimens are likely to cause false negative results.

## Specimen processing

*Microscopy*

Gram stain of a carefully obtained specimen can provide a rapid presumptive diagnosis of:

- urethritis
- cervicitis
- vaginal discharge.

Complementary microscopic methods include direct wet preparations and immunofluorescent techniques used in the diagnosis of vaginal discharge and genital ulcer. If performed in the clinic, these simple tests can have an immediate impact on management of the patient's infection.

*Gram negative diplococci* This finding inside neutrophils in urethral exudate from a male patient is highly predictive of gonococcal infection. Around 90% males with gonorrhoea will be smear positive. Although Gram stain should be performed on endocervical swabs, a negative result is less conclusive, since only 60% with gonococcal cervicitis will be positive on smear.

*Graded Gram stain* This is the method of choice for diagnosis of bacterial vaginosis, and has replaced the former method involving the KOH 'whiff' test, a search for 'clue' cells and culture for *Gardnerella vaginalis*. Graded Gram stain requires scoring for the absence of Gram positive bacilli, and the presence of both Gram negative coccobacilli and Gram negative spiral bacilli (details in Nugent RP et al 1991 J Clin Microbiol 29: 297–301). If this method is used, *G. vaginalis* culture can be dispensed with.

*Gram stain or an unstained coverslip preparation* This can be used to look for yeasts in possible cases of vaginal candidiasis. A direct preparation is more reliable than culture, since low numbers of *C. albicans* can be present as members of the indigenous vaginal flora.

*Exudate from the base of a genital ulcer* This should be Gram stained for the 'school of fish' Gram negative bacilli of chancroid, especially if the ulcer is painful and does not have an indurated edge. If the ulcer is painless and has an indurated edge, primary syphilis is more likely and an unstained coverslip preparation should be examined for spirochaetes. It takes experience to be able to distinguish possible *Treponema pallidum* from commensal spirochaetes present on some patients. To avoid this problem, a modified version of the fluorescent treponemal antibody test can be applied to a heat-fixed sample on an unstained glass slide. *Trichomonas vaginalis* is best seen in an unstained coverslip preparation of vaginal exudate.

### Culture

As the clinical features of gonococcal infection are indistinguishable from those of chlamydial infection, an attempt should be made to culture both species from genital exudate specimens.

Most laboratories will use a selective medium for *N. gonorrhoeae* to exclude skin, gastrointestinal and vaginal commensal species. Some media (e.g. VCNT) may inhibit the growth of a proportion of gonococci. Cell culture is more sensitive than direct immunofluorescent methods of detecting *Chlamydia pneumoniae* from genital sites, particularly if a second

---

**Remember:**

- Herpes simplex virus is prone to deteriorate during transport. Viral culture should be started shortly after specimen collection to guarantee a high probability of virus recovery.
- Isolation of small numbers of yeasts from vaginal swabs is less reliable an indicator of candidiasis than the presence of yeasts and leukocytes on direct Gram stain of vaginal exudate.
- The isolation of *Gardnerella vaginalis* per se is not necessarily diagnostic of bacterial vaginosis. Graded evaluation of Gram stained exudate is more reliable.

pass culture is made from each clinical specimen. It is also less prone to false positive results. Exudate suspended in transport medium or urine should be centrifuged onto cell monolayers which are then treated with cyclophosphamide before incubation.

## Reporting results

In order to preserve patient confidentiality, the presence of a specific sexually transmitted pathogen in a patient's specimen should be communicated to persons outside the diagnostic laboratory with great care. No such result should be faxed or given over the phone unless you can be certain that it will reach the intended recipient **and no-one else**. Failure to follow these simple precautions may result in potentialy avoidable litigation.

## Presumptive therapy

The patient should be referred to a genitourinary medicine clinic where his or her infection(s) can be managed confidentially, and contact tracing facilities are available.

Presumptive therapy will be a variation on the following:

### Urethral, cervical gonorrhoea

- Amoxycillin 3.0 g and probenicid 1.0 g p.o.
- Spectinomycin 2.0 g i.m. if PPNG suspected.

### Urethral, cervical chlamydial infection

- Tetracycline 500 mg p.o. qds × 7d.
- Doxycycline 200 mg p.o. bd × 7d.

### Vaginal discharge

- Trichomoniasis: metronidazole 2 mg p.o. single dose.
- Candidiasis: topical imidazole × 3 d or fluconazole 150 mg p.o. single dose.
- Bacterial vaginosis: metronidazole 500 mg bd × 7 d or metronidazole 2 g p.o. single dose.

### Genital ulcer

- Primary syphilis: procaine penicillin 600 mg i.m. daily × 10 d.
- Penicillin allergy: tetracycline 500 mg p.o. qds × 15 d.
- Herpes: acyclovir 200 mg p.o. × 5 per day × 5 d.
- Chancroid: ceftriaxone 250 mg i.m. single dose.

## Contact tracing

In the UK there is a statutory requirement to trace the sexual contacts of patients with specified genitourinary infections, i.e. gonorrhoea, syphilis and chlamydial infection. The principal reason for contact tracing is to prevent further spread of infection in the sexually active population, but treatment of contacts of the index case will also help prevent reinfection.

Other infections for which contacts may be sought include genital herpes and genital warts.

The preferred method is to get the index patient to advise all recent sexual contacts to attend a genitourinary medicine clinic. If the patient is reluctant to do this, an anonymous letter advising the need for a confidential consultation can be sent providing names and addresses have been given by the patient. Contact tracers have the legal authority to visit named contacts, but in many areas staff may be concerned to avoid breaching patient confidentiality or risking assault.

# INFECTIVE ENDOCARDITIS

## Treatment

*Fully sensitive viridans group streptococci*

- Benzyl penicillin 1.8 g (3Mu) every 4 h i.v. and gentamicin 80 mg every 12 h i.v. for 2 wk.
- Then amoxycillin 500 mg–1 g every 8 hours for 2 wk.

 The risk of gentamicin toxicity may outweigh the benefits of use unless careful monitoring of levels is carried out. The alternative is to continue high dose benzyl penicillin i.v. for 4 weeks.

*Resistant viridans group streptococci*

- Benzyl penicillin and gentamicin i.v. as above for 4 wk.

*Penicillin hypersensitivity*

- Vancomycin by i.v. infusion.
- Some recommend adding gentamicin, but toxicity is a problem.

## Prophylaxis of endocarditis

Patients at increased risk of infective endocarditis are those with prosthetic valves, patent ductus arteriosus, ventriculoseptal defect, left-side mitral or aortic valve disease, aortic coarctation and a previous episode of endocarditis. There is no significant risk in atrial septal defect, cardiac pacemaker, coronary heart disease.

Procedures that result in a high risk of subsequent endocarditis are dental extraction or scaling, and operative procedures on the gastrointestinal or genitourinary tract.

The following is an outline of guidelines for antibiotic prophylaxis of endocarditis for patients at increased risk (above):

*Dental procedures, ENT surgery*

- Amoxycillin p.o. 1 h before procedure, or
- Erythromycin stearate 1.5 g 1 h before, 0.5 g 6 h later.

*General anaesthesia for high risk procedure*

- Amoxycillin 1 g i.m. just before induction, 0.5 g 6 h later, or
- Amoxycillin 3 g p.o. 4 h before surgery, 3 g p.o. post operation.

*Penicillin allergy or penicillin therapy in previous month*

- Vancomycin 1 g i.v. infusion over 60 min, then
- Gentamicin 120 mg i.v. just before induction.

*Genitourinary procedures*

- Amoxycillin and gentamicin to address risk of enterococci; if UTI, extend cover for urinary isolate.

*Obstetric and gynaecological procedures*

- Prophylaxis only if prosthetic valve.

## PERICARDITIS

Pericardial fluid is a rare specimen, usually obtained by a cardiothoracic surgeon. If there is opportunity to control timing, thoracocentesis should be done during working hours, and the specimen transferred to the laboratory immediately.

Cytology (total and differential WCC), Gram stain and culture should be carried out as for other normally sterile fluids. Mycobacterial media and cooked meat broth should be inoculated. Culture for enteroviruses should also be set up. If tuberculous pericarditis is a possible diagnosis, a biopsy should be taken while the opportunity exists. If a fungal infection is possible, silver stain will be required.

### Treatment

● Purulent pericarditis: 4–6 weeks, according to Gram and culture.
● Tuberculous: 2 years with 3 agents (e.g. RIP) plus steroids.

# PERITONITIS

Peritonitis following damage to or leakage from abdominal viscus results in spillage of intestinal contents. Pathogens will usually be mixed intestinal flora. Paracentesis is rarely useful in tuberculous peritonitis. Patients with Tenchkoff catheter for peritoneal dialysis are at risk of infection via the lumen or tracking alongside the catheter.

### Diagnostic criteria for CAPD peritonitis

At least two of the following conditions:

- cloudy effluent: >100 leucocytes/mm³
- abdominal pain
- organisms in effluent.

### Procedure

Obtain at least 30 ml effluent after careful disinfection of sampling port with alcohol.

### Specimen processing

Obtain a total leucocyte count using counting chamber. Spin 10 ml to obtain deposit for Gram stain and differential count. Filter remaining 20 ml of peritoneal dialysate via sterile 0.45 µm Millipore filter for aerobic and anaerobic culture. Any further effluent can be inoculated into blood culture bottles.

### Troubleshooting

Negative culture but evidence of peritonitis means:

- early morning effluent (higher WCC)
- very low organism count
- intra-abdominal pathology: cholecystitis, appendicitis etc
- bleeding due to menstruation, ovulation
- eosinophilic peritonitis — reaction to dialysis equipment
- unusual organisms — mycobacteria, fungi, parasites.

### Follow-up

A ward visit to pass on preliminary culture results is an opportunity to check presumptive therapy is appropriate, review the initial response to therapy and encourage the physicians to remove the catheter if indicated.

### Presumptive therapy

- Intraperitoneal vancomycin and aminoglycoside given in bag of dialysis fluid.
- Add rifampicin if relapsing *S. aureus* infection.

## Indications for removing Tenchkoff catheter

- Gangrenous or perforated viscus.
- Fungal, yeast, mycobacterial or *Pseudomonas* infection.

# PLEURAL EFFUSION

Around 40% pneumonias result in formation of a pleural effusion. A pleural tap should be considered under the following circumstances:

- Reason for effusion is not clear.
- > 10 mm effusion shadow on lateral CXR.
- Persistent effusion despite therapy.
- Increasing size of effusion.
- Evidence of loculation.

## Specimen processing

- Total leucocyte count (if thick, dilute in 1/10 isotonic saline).
- Centrifuge.
- Prepare Gram stain and differential count from deposit.
- Inoculate media for culture.

## Troubleshooting

- A differential count is more useful than a total leucocyte count.
- Bizarre cells should be referred to cytologist.
- If lymphocytes predominate, this may indicate tuberculosis — TB sometimes causes eosinophilic effusion. If considering TB, sub to mycobacterial media and advise pleural biopsy (higher yield).
- pH < 7.0 may indicate a complicated effusion needing drainage.

## Follow-up

Results of cytology and Gram stain provide an opportunity to find out more about the patient's condition, and the range of diagnoses being considered. If clinical features and these preliminary results suggest a pneumococcal infection, blood culture should be arranged. The start of antimicrobial therapy should not wait for culture results; presumptive therapy should be commenced on the basis of the Gram stain. Modifications can be made to the initial therapy on the basis of culture and susceptibility results.

# RESPIRATORY INFECTIONS

The potential for contamination of respiratory specimens by the indigenous flora of the mouth, nasopharynx and oropharynx makes interpretation of culture results a problem. Care and attention must therefore be paid to specimen collection for both throat swabs and expectorated sputum. Poor specimens are more likely to produce uninterpretable results.

A wide range of respiratory pathogens may be encountered, but not all can be sought for. The requesting clinician must attempt to narrow down the list of potentials to a shortlist based on the working diagnosis. It must also be recognised that, unless otherwise directed, only the more common and easily recovered pathogens will be sought for.

## SUSPECTED PNEUMONIA

**Remember:**
- a rapid aetiological diagnosis is rarely made
- a very wide range of pathogens is possible
- there is a correspondingly wide range of antibiotics.

### History
Helpful points in the history are: age, date of hospital admission.

### Physical examination
Key features to look for are: rashes, petechiae (viral infection, or septicaemia) and pleural effusion.

### General investigations
- Peripheral white cell count: > 15 000/mm³ and left shift in bacterial pneumonia; most viral infections have a normal count.
- Chest X-ray: main role is to discover extent of consolidation. Look for:
  — consolidation: lobar/segmental, broncho-, interstitial, cavitating
  — presence of pleural effusion.

 Chest X-ray features are rarely pathognomic of a specific microbial aetiology, though they may provide some useful clues.

*Specimens other than sputum*

- Blood culture: good chance of positive in untreated, early lobar pneumonia.
- Pleural fluid (cell count/differential, Gram stain, culture):
  — if present, a good way of avoiding problem of contamination by oral bacteria
  — bacteria present on Gram stain are always significant
  — neutrophils usually signify bacterial infection.
- Cerebrospinal fluid: if any suspicion of concomitant meningitis.

*Invasive diagnostic procedures*

- Specialist laboratory experience may not be available without prior arrangement.
- These are generally discouraged after normal laboratory hours when a full range of lab tests is not available. Specimens deteriorate quickly (within a few hours) and may be unsuitable for microscopy by the time the laboratory reopens.
- Do not confuse bronchoscopic lavage/bronchoalveolar lavage with salivary specimen and discard as unsuitable.
- Percutaneous thoracotomy (PCT), bronchoscopic biopsy, and open lung biopsy all have specific uses in the diagnosis of infections in immunocompromised patients, and carry a small risk of pneumothorax.

## Epidemiological clues

Physicians rely heavily on the initial clinical picture to help with preliminary therapeutic decisions by narrowing the range of possible pathogens. There is considerable overlap in both the range of clinical presentation and the microbial species that cause them. Textbook descriptions of typical clinical presentations may be based on the later stages of a condition, or a collection of features from epidemiological studies.

Certain signs and symptoms provide clues to the causative organism:

- Fever, productive cough with rusty sputum, sudden onset pleuritic chest pain, possibly a cold sore or shingles, and lobar consolidation — consider *Streptococcus pneumoniae*.
- Pharyngitis, a nonproductive cough, a young adult with family contacts, ambulant despite chest X-ray changes — consider *Mycoplasma pneumoniae*.
- A nonproductive cough, with confusion and diarrhoea in a middle-aged smoker, possibly with a history of recent airconditioner or hotel shower exposure — consider *Legionella pneumophila*.
- Fever and productive cough following epidemic pneumonia, possibly with pneumatocoele on chest X-ray — consider *Staphylococcus aureus*.

- Fever and productive cough in a smoker with a history of chronic lung disease, and patchy consolidation on chest X-ray — consider *Streptococcus pneumoniae* and/or *Haemophilus influenzae*.
- Fever, productive cough and haemoptysis, with recent weight loss, hilar lymphadenopathy and apical consolidation — consider *Mycobacterium tuberculosis*.
- Fever and productive cough, with thick, viscous, red sputum, and history of alcohol dependency — consider *Klebsiella pneumoniae*.
- Fever and progressive breathlessness in HIV+ patient or transplant recipient — consider *Pneumocystis carinii*.
- Nonproductive cough, fever and patchy, interstitial consolidation with history of recent exposure to parrot or similar bird — consider *Chlamydia psittaci*.

## Presumptive therapy

*Community-acquired lobar pneumonia* 1.8 g benzyl penicillin i.v. every 4 h, or 300 mg procaine penicillin 12 h (add cefotaxime if history of chronic lung disease).

*Atypical pneumonia* 500–1000 mg erythromycin i.v. 6 h (add rifampicin for older adult if severely ill on admission); alternative is tetracycline.

*Community-acquired bronchopneumonia* Ampicillin or erythromycin, by i.v. route if $O_2$ required.

*Aspiration pneumonia or abscess* Clindamycin i.v. (superior to metronidazole); alternative is benzyl penicillin in high dose.

*Hospital-acquired pneumonia* Choice should be directed towards *Staphylococcus aureus* and Gram negative bacilli including *Pseudomonas aeruginosa*, but will depend heavily on local susceptibility patterns.

*Acute pulmonary tuberculosis* Rifampicin, isoniazid and pyrazinamide (remember to apply additional infection control precautions, and ask if HIV status known).

*Acute bronchitis in children < 5 years* Nebulised ribavirin may be valuable if the child needs to be in hospital, but is not yet in need of mechanical ventilation.

## Specimen collection

*Throat swab* Needs a tongue depressor or similar to help avoid contact with buccal mucosa and tongue. Posterior oropharynx should be swabbed. If *N. gonorrhoeae* is suspected, use charcoal swab.

- If epiglottitis suspected do not attempt to swab an awake child without first installing an airway (4-fold increase in mortality if obstructed airway).
- Other specimens to think about: blood culture, and urine for Hib antigen detection.

*Pernasal swab* **for B. pertussis** Dacron or alginate tipped swab should be passed along the inferior surface of the nasopharynx, backwards as far as it will go. Then swab to selective bordetella medium at bedside. The highest isolation rate is in the first 2–3 weeks of the infection.

*Sputum* Most patients need coaching in how to cough up 'phlegm' from deep in the chest, and propel it into a suitable wide-mouthed container; otherwise they will spit out little sputum and much saliva. A physiotherapist is usually the best person to supervise. It may help to get the patient to wash out the mouth with sterile water first.

*Bronchoalveolar lavage* Respiratory material obtained via bronchoscope should be clearly labelled ('BAL') to avoid discarding as saliva. Unless double lumen, or plug-tipped, deep BAL specimens are still prone to some contamination by upper respiratory flora.

*Invasive specimens* Thoracocentesis, transtracheal aspirate, lung puncture and open lung biopsy should all be clearly labelled and may justify liaison between requesting clinician and lab prior to collection in order to arrange special investigations.

## Mandatory culture-based procedures

### Throat swab
Blood agar for β haemolytic streptococci, groups A, C and G (sheep blood agar, with coverslip over 1° inoculum, incubated 48 h to enhance oxygen labile haemolysis).

### Sputum

- Blood agar with optichin disk in 2° streak, and chocolate agar incubated in 5% $CO_2$ for *S. pneumoniae, H. influenzae, S. aureus* and *Ps. aeruginosa*.
- Hospital patients; MacConkey agar for Enterobacteriaceae.

## Discretionary procedures

### Throat swab

*Yeasts* Sabouraud's agar if oral thrush is suspected. Confirmation is by germ tube test, chlamydospore production or substrate utilisation.

*N. gonorrhoeae* VCAT or similar agar if STD clinic, or if clinical details suggestive. Confirmation is by CTA sugar utilisation tests or equivalent.

*B. pertussis* Cephalexin-charcoal agar if pernasal swab is submitted. (CCA has longer shelf life than Bordet–Gengou agar). Confirmation is by latex agglutination.

*C. diphtheriae* Tellurite agar if diphtheria is strongly suspected. Confirmation is by colonial, microscopic appearance and sugar reactions. Toxin production is confirmed by agar incorporation ELEK test.

### Lower respiratory

*Mycoplasma pneumoniae* Takes 10–14 d to grow on mycoplasma agar, is difficult to see and requires neutralisation of substrate for confirmation. Specific diagnosis is usually by CFT (18–21 d interval to convalescent serum) or IgM EIA 7–10 d post onset.

*Legionella spp* Usually are not seen on sputum Gram stain. They grow on BCYE agar after 48–72 h, giving colonies with a ground glass appearance. Direct fluorescent antigen test on sputum smear is prone to variable interpretation. Serodiagnosis is by IF or ELISA. Urine antigen detection may also be available.

*Chlamydia spp* Isolation is not normally attempted for respiratory infection. Retrospective serological diagnosis is by chlamydia CFT (only genus specific; species is deduced by the pattern of response to range of antigens shared by members of genus).

*Mycobacterium tuberculosis* Culture sputum after treatment (decontamination to remove commensal and other non mycobacteria) on Lowenstein–Jensen or similar media in any cases of suspected pulmonary tuberculosis.

*Pneumocystis carinii* Best specimen is open lung biopsy but highly invasive. BAL is best compromise. Induced sputum is highly variable; it depends on skill and compliance of the patient. Immunofluorescent antigen labelling procedure is specific but very labour-intensive. Quicker procedures are: Toluidine blue or Grocott's stains for cysts, Geimsa for trophozoites.

*Respiratory syncytial virus* Rapid diagnosis is possible by immunofluorescence on nasal washings (best) or respiratory secretions. Place specimen in transport medium and rush to lab on wet ice. Antigen capture ELISA is less sensitive.

*Other respiratory viruses (adeno-, influenza, parainfluenza viruses)* Use serum for retrospective serological diagnosis.

### Sputum microscopy (→ Table 1.10)

Gram stains containing >15 squamous epithelial cells per low power field (or < 25 neutrophils per LPF, in non-neutropoenic patient) should be rejected as unsuitable for further examination. Neutrophils and > 10 Gram positive diplococci per high power field are strongly suggestive of pneumococcal infection.

If there are any grounds for suspecting pulmonary tuberculosis do an acid fast stain as well: either Zeihl–Neelsen or auramine-phenol.

---

**TABLE 1.10  Stains for sputum microscopy**

**Gram stain:** thin film at low power (×100). Take an average of 5 fields worth of epithelial cells and neutrophils; take care to note whether patient is neutropoenic

| Cells/h.p.f. | Report as |
|---|---|
| 0 | 0 |
| <10 | ± |
| 10–25 | + |
| >25 | ++ |

**Ziehl–Neelsen stain:** thin film, heat fixed, examined at high power (×1000)

| A.F.B. | Report as |
|---|---|
| 0 in 300 fields | – |
| 1–2 per 300 fields | ± |
| 1–10 per 100 fields | + |
| 1–10 per 10 fields | ++ |
| 1–10 per fields | +++ |
| 10 per field | ++++ |

An equivocal result (e.g. a single doubtful bacillus) obtained on-call should be left until normal lab hours for repeat stain and confirmation. Acid fast bacilli may be found more quickly on Z-N in strongly positive smears by finding clusters of neutrophils under low power, then moving to the oil immersion lens.

---

### Safety

All lower respiratory specimens should be handled in a biological safety cabinet (class I) in a category 3 laboratory. Disposable gloves should be worn. Disposable loops should be used. The bunsen burner should be shielded if used at all, or a hot plate used instead. Centrifuge buckets should be sealable.

### Interpretation of culture results

#### Throat swabs

- *S. pyogenes* may be present in small numbers (minority of organisms present or < + growth) as a harmless commensal. However +++ or pure growth should always be regarded as significant. Haemolysis may not be prominent, if incubated aerobically for only 24 h or on horse blood agar.

- *Arcanobacterium haemolyticum* and *Corynebacterium ureae* may be spotted if you are really determined, but these are probably missed most of the time.

### Sputum

Remember that both *S. pneumoniae* and *H. influenzae* are occasional members of the indigenous flora of the upper respiratory tract. However, pure or +++ predominant growth should not be dismissed as insignificant. The optichin disk will help you to spot *S. pneumoniae*, and a staph streak, if used, may help with *H. influenzae* as will the characteristic smell of indole. Confirmatory tests must always be completed before issuing a report.

- *Branhamella catarrhalis* should only be reported as significant and tested against antibiotics if intracellular Gram negative cocci have been observed on the sputum Gram stain.
- *S. aureus* may pose a problem, but should always be treated as potentially significant during an influenza epidemic, when there is a cavitating pneumonia, and in hospital patients with suspected nosocomial pneumonia (commonest Gram positive cause of NP).
- *Pseudomonas aeruginosa* produces fuzzy grey-green colonies with a mouldy hay smell and also poses a problem: it may be a minority organism that has overgrown the others during prolonged transit. But it may also be the cause of nosocomial pneumonia or exacerbation of cystic fibrosis.
- *Nocardia* and actinomycetes take a long time to grow: *Nocardia* sp. grows aerobically on blood agar, and actinomycetes anaerobically. You will probably only pick these up if you are looking for them in high risk patients, e.g. renal transplant.
- *Aspergillus fumigatus* often appears on sputum culture plates as an airborne contaminant, and sometimes as a result of pulmonary disease. Invasive aspergillosis is better diagnosed by biopsy, and allergic disease by demonstrating serum precipitins.

### Therapeutic issues

#### Pharyngitis

Pharyngitis caused by group A streptococci can proceed to rheumatic fever. Penicillin is the only agent shown to prevent RF but it must either be given orally for 10 days or as a single i.m. dose of benzathine penicillin. But, provided therapy starts within one week of onset, it will still have a preventive effect. So it is possible to wait for culture results before commencing penicillin therapy for streptococcal pharyngitis. Direct antigen testing can help speed up start of therapy, but negative results must still be confirmed by culture.

#### Pneumonia

See presumptive therapy, above. Antimicrobial therapy is not usually required in acute bronchitis in adults or acute aspiration (Mendelsson's syndrome).

### Bronchiolitis
If resulting in hospital admission, this will often be caused by RSV. Mainstay of management is oxygen, clearance of respiratory secretions, and adequate hydration. Use of ribavirin is controversial, but severe or complicated cases may benefit if ribavirin therapy is started early.

### Pertussis
Infants (< 1 yr) are at greatest risk of complications. Steroids or salbutamol can reduce the severity of paroxysms. Erythromycin is given for 2 weeks. It does not benefit the patient much unless started in the early catarrhal stage, but helps reduce infectivity (siblings etc.) 5 days after start of course.

### Pulmonary tuberculosis
Best results are achieved with short-course, 4-agent regimens, using the directly observed approach to therapy to ensure compliance. Failure to do so can result in community and even hospital outbreaks of multidrug resistant TB. Treatment of PTB should therefore be supervised by a chest physician with special interest in TB.

## Follow-up
Streptococcal pharyngitis in any inpatient healthcare setting can lead to serious hospital-acquired infection. Patients with this infection must be drawn to the attention of infection control staff. Hospital staff working in operating theatre or otherwise liable to transmit their infection to vulnerable patients should be excused duties until free of group A streptococci, usually at least 48 h after starting treatment.

Pneumonias often take longer to respond radiologically than clinical signs suggest. Treatment should not be judged to have failed because the X-ray hasn't confirmed the patient's apparent clinical improvement. Conversely, pneumonia remains a disease with a high mortality, despite optimal treatment; some patients will continue to deteriorate despite heroic efforts to prevent the inevitable. Do not overestimate the contribution sputum microscopy and culture make to the patient's acute management. Remember that the requesting clinician may only be confused by laboratory reports listing several potential pathogens and a plethora of antibiotic sensitivity results.

*B. pertussis*, mycobacteria and RSV all have implications for infection control. Positive results need to be communicated to infection control staff immediately so that additional precautions can be instituted straight away.

# SEPTICAEMIA

Blood culture is the single most important microbiological investigation in septicaemia. However, additional specimens should be collected from any identifiable focus of infection. Non-microbiological specimens will be required to test the following:

- urea and electrolytes; renal function
- blood gases
- clotting function and FDPs, DIC.

## Setting up a blood culture

---

**Procedure**
1. Do not rush; avoid risk of needlestick or contamination.
2. Disinfect bottle tops with isopropyl alcohol; leave to dry.
3. Disinfect venesection site after palpation, with alcohol and iodophor, following a widening spiral pattern.
4. Collect sufficient blood for culture and other investigations.
5. Dispense into culture bottle, without changing needles.
6. Clean iodophor from venesection site with alcohol.
7. Arrange dispatch of culture set and request form.

---

### Volume

The single most important determinant of positive blood culture results. Use:

- 5–10 ml/bottle for adult patients
- 1–2 ml/bottle for infants
- but note high volume bottles for some automated systems (optimal fill usually indicated on bottle).

If a smaller than recommended volume of blood is obtained, fill fewer bottles. Do not overfill, or both constituents will be diluted past optimal concentration.

### Number

For a single febrile episode: 2–3 sets (pairs) are usually adequate. A positive result after more than 4 sets is very rare.

### Timing

In most emergency settings, take 2–3 sets from different sites over 1 h. Cultures should be timed, if possible, to coincide with temperature peak. If the presumed source of bacteraemia is vascular, timing is less crucial as bacterial count is likely to be more constant.

## Getting it to the lab

To avoid losing valuable blood cultures between the point of collection and the laboratory, make sure that the staff sending them know how to get them to you. Procedures vary considerably between hospitals, depending on variables such as out-of-hours portering, proximity of the lab and automation of blood culture analysis.

It is important to ensure that:

- bottles are correctly and carefully labelled and accompanied by a matching request form
- blood cultures are not refrigerated
- if storage or lengthy transit cannot be avoided, bottles are kept at room temperature.

Some hospitals working with a manual blood culture procedure provide a holding incubator for out-of-hours blood cultures. This system cannot be used with newer automated analysers (such as BacTAlert or Bactec 9240) where delayed entry may result in false negative results.

## Preliminary blood culture results

### Out-of-hours positives

- Inspect the second member of a possible positive culture set and any other sets submitted at or around the same time.
- Check in the daybook or computer record for any previous work on the same cultures sets.
- A positive result should prompt a search for results on any other specimens submitted at or around the same time.

### Detection of positives: manual system

All blood culture bottles should be inspected at least once out of hours every day, to shorten time to detection. Even if all bottles are to be routinely subcultured onto solid media, possible positives should be singled out and given priority. Look for:

- turbidity
- haemolysis
- visible growth (especially on top of blood layer).

If detection alert devices are used, you should still inspect the main chamber of the bottle. All possible positives should be:

- Gram stained
- subcultured onto nonselective solid media

- incubated according to standard protocol
- set up for direct antimicrobial susceptibility testing if bacteria seen.

*With Gram negative bacilli* in high concentration, try oxidase test on supernatant. With possible *S. pneumoniae*, try bile solubility test on supernatant.

### Detection of positives: automated blood culture analysers

Newer machines will produce a preliminary result within 24 h of the blood culture arriving in the laboratory. In exceptional circumstances, processing time may be as little as 3 h. These rapid processing times will only be passed on to the ward, and benefit the patient, if the laboratory is open to receive blood cultures and report positives around the clock. That means the blood culture analyser will dictate the organisation of out-of-hours work; it is only justifiable if ward staff are willing and able to act on your results. If not, a batch processing system will be followed.

A positive result (growth value, growth index, printout, alarm, etc.) needs confirmation by Gram stain. Then follow sequence described in Manual system, above.

## Reporting your result

Blood culture results are amongst the most important the diagnostic lab produces. They must be communicated accurately to staff looking after the patient as soon as possible.

1. Locate the patient:
   - written on request form
   - ward/unit written on bottle
   - patient register
   - bleep requesting doctor.
2. Speak to the most senior nurse on ward.
3. Dictate patient's identification, time/date of culture and laboratory observations. If names of pathogens are communicated, make sure they are spelled correctly.
4. Try to find out about the patient's progress, current antibiotic therapy, and the identity of on-call medical staff responsible for the patient.
5. Contact the duty medical officer to discuss significance of results, and any necessary alteration to therapy.
6. Note time of verbal report, name of staff spoken to and what was said, for future reference.

 **Be persistent if you cannot locate the patient or any doctor who will accept responsibility for the patient.**

## Follow-up

Any preliminary work done on positive blood cultures out-of-hours should be followed up the next morning.

- Go over the results of the Gram stain.
- Check agar plates for early signs of growth.
- Examine direct ST plates.
- Look again for any other results from the same patient.
- If necessary, get the relevant MLSO and record clerk to help; visit the patient, review history, results of other investigations and check treatment chart.

Decide if appropriate action was taken, and whether it needs modification. If so, locate the medical staff responsible for the patient (junior staff appreciate having up-to-date results for the ward round). Discuss the results and their significance with the most senior doctor available. If changes to therapy are required, encourage, propose or suggest, but do not be overly critical; you do not have the final responsibility for the clinical outcome. Ask if it would be useful to make a note of these preliminary results in the patient's record, but be brief: stick to the results as observed in the lab, with the barest of comments on their significance, unless a consultant has requested a formal clinical consultation (in which case specific clinical issues will have to be addressed).

Results of susceptibility testing will often come through on the second day or later, providing a further opportunity to visit the patient and assess progress. By this time the microbiology service will probably be intimately involved in a multidisciplinary effort if the patient has failed to make a rapid response. It is therefore worth ensuring that one medical microbiologist is responsible for co-ordinating all the laboratory's work on the patient.

Further cultures are only really necessary in case of:

- a further septic episode
- infective endocarditis, where initial cultures were negative.

# SEPTIC ARTHRITIS

> ● An effusion in a hot joint is not always due to infection.
> ● Infection of the joint does not necessarily result in a purulent effusion.

## Specimen processing

● Total WCC (may need dilution in 1/10 isotonic saline).
● Microscopy in polarising light.
● Spun deposit:
  — Gram stain
  — differential WCC
  — culture for bacteria including *S. aureus*, streptococci, enterobacteriaceae and *H. influenzae* (in children).

## Troubleshooting

● Sterile leucocytosis: acute RA, crystal synovitis.
● Other infections to think of: mycobacteria (biopsy needed)
  — gonococcal infection (DGI)
  — viruses (e.g. rubella)
  — fungi (e.g. *Sporothrix*).

## Presumptive therapy

● Young children: cefotaxime i.v. t.d.s. × 2 wk.
● Adults/children < 5 yr, GPC in clusters: cloxacillin i.v. × 3 wk.
● Adults, GPC in chains: penicillin i.v. × 2 wk.
● Adults with DGI: penicillin i.v. or ceftriaxone.

## Follow-up

The cytological and Gram stain results need to be backed up with specific information about the patient's age, any history of joint disease and, in adults, sexual habits. By the time culture results are ready there may also be a blood culture result to tie up with synovial fluid cultures. This may be a good time to encourage rationalisation of antimicrobial therapy, or if necessary push for further investigations in culture negative patients.

# SOFT TISSUE INFECTIONS

Specimens from soft tissue sites are prone to contamination by superficial skin flora or temporary commensals. Attention to specimen collection technique and interpretation of culture results is required to ensure clinically relevant laboratory reports.

## Clinical presentation

The majority of soft tissue infections the laboratory has any dealing with will be superficial surgical wound infections. Other major categories of soft tissue infection include:

- infections of the skin appendages
- superficial/spreading infections
- deep soft tissue infection,
- infections associated with specific occupational or geographical exposure.

The clinical history and structures involved are obviously important in naming the clinical syndrome, but there is continued debate of classification of infections in the deeper soft tissues. This reflects the overlap between the overt clinical and histological consequences of infection with the more common pathogens. One species can cause a variety of presentations. Conversely, one type of clinical entity can be caused by a variety of species. Indeed, more than a single bacterial species may be involved.

Recent media attention on necrotising fasciitis has made doctors more aware of the difficulties of arriving at a confident working diagnosis early in the management of the condition, when there is still time to arrest the spread of infection. If in doubt, an early surgical opinion should be sought, and radical debridement considered.

In patients with deep soft tissue infection, the onset of the following clinical features may indicate a worsening prognosis:

- clinically apparent crepitus
- deep pain in affected tissues
- fever
- tachycardia
- tachypnoea
- confusion
- cyanosis.

## Specimen collection

Nonsterile sites such as the skin surface should be cleaned prior to specimen collection. It is less than satisfactory to pass a dry cotton-tipped swab gently over a wound surface without prior cleansing. This will often cause the patient some discomfort, but that may be necessary to avoid misleading laboratory results. If there is a lot of pus it should be sent in a sterile container, rather than on a swab.

The entry points of orthopaedic pins or surgical drains are often heavily colonised with bacteria. These should not be swabbed unless there is evidence of severe or rapidly spreading local inflammation. A different sampling approach must be used if there is any suspicion of infection in deeper tissues.

Spreading erythema without a purulent inflammatory exudate, crusting or vesicles, can sometimes be sampled by instilling a small quantity of sterile water (without preservatives) intradermally at the advancing edge, and reaspirating into a small syringe (fine needle aspiration; FNA). The syringe and needle should be taken directly to the laboratory for immediate processing, and to avoid needlestick injury. Vesicle and blister fluid can be aspirated into a syringe for subsequent processing but, if a vesicular eruption could be due to viral infection, a fine-tipped swab should be rubbed over the base of a vesicle to dislodge epithelial cells, and then placed in viral transport medium.

If deep soft tissue infection is suspected, the patient probably needs an early surgical opinion. Surgical debridement is an excellent opportunity to obtain a high quality specimen from a normally sterile site. This should be treated as an urgent specimen if the patient shows any constitutional signs of systemic infection or rapid progression of a local lesion. Make sure the referring clinician takes personal responsibility for getting the specimen to the laboratory, especially if an operative procedure is to be performed out-of-hours. But also ensure that the results of Gram stain are followed through with a return call or visit. These patients may also require blood cultures, culture of abscess contents, blister/vesicle fluid or needle aspirate from a spreading edge.

Chronic soft tissue infections should be biopsied and treated with special stains for unusual pathogens such as mycobacteria, actinomycetes, *Nocardia* spp. and *Sporothrix schenkii*.

## Specimen processing

### Microscopy

Some laboratories do not perform Gram stains on all wound swabs, because of the mixture of bacterial species that can colonise surface sites. While it may be appropriate to follow this policy with the relatively low priority, routine surgical wound swabs, high priority specimens from severely ill patients and all specimens from normally sterile, deep sites should be Gram stained.

Take care not to make the smear too thick, otherwise the stain may lift off the glass or crack before examination.

- Neutropoenic patients may not have detectable neutrophils in inflammatory exudate.
- The exudate formed in clostridial myonecrosis is thin and may lack neutrophils. The bacilli seen in acute disease do not usually have visible spores.
- Microscopy of clinical specimens plays no role in the acute diagnosis of tetanus.

Pus from patients with suspected actinomycosis should be squashed between a glass slide and a coverslip, before Gram staining. This will make the tangle of branching Gram positive bacilli in 'sulphur granules' easier to see.

Vesicle fluid should be examined for viral pathogens under the electron microscope.

Skin scrapings, hair or nail clippings for dermatophytes (see Fig. 1.5) should be treated with KOH to disperse keratin and examined for fungal hyphae. Do not try to name the species, but wait for lactophenol cotton blue preparation of cultures.

### Culture

Mandatory procedures for all soft tissue specimens include culture on blood agar aerobically, anaerobically, and on MacConkey aerobically.

Discretionary procedures include culture on haemolysed (chocolate) blood agar aerobically, with $CO_2$ and microaerophilically, culture on Sabouraud's agar (or alternative solid mycology media), and antibiotic containing anaerobic agar. Any evidence to suggest chronic soft tissue infection other than dermatophytosis should lead to prolonged incubation for fastidious anaerobes, actinomycetes and other higher bacteria and culture for mycobacteria and unusual fungal species.

### Interpretation

The most common bacterial pathogen isolated from surgical wound infections is *S. aureus*. Some of these isolates may be no more than secondary colonisers of a damaged skin surface, but if sufficient clinical information has been given, it has to be assumed that the patient may require specific antistaphylococcal therapy.

There is less difficulty interpreting the presence of *Streptococcus pyogenes* in a wound swab, or specimen from another soft tissue infection, and anaerobic species are usually important from a carefully taken specimen. However, *Pseudomonas aeruginosa*, *Proteus* and other Enterobacteriaceae and Enterococci are usually present as innocent bystanders, especially when the specimen comes from a large epidermal defect such as a venous stasis ulcer

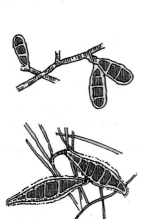

***Epidermophyton floccosum***
Club-shaped macroconidia, 3–4 cells,
no microconidia

***Microsporum canis***
Asymetrical, spindle-shaped macroconidia
with rough wall

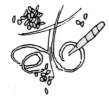

***Trichophyton mentagrophytes***
Occasional sausage-shaped macronidia,
many micronidia in clusters; spiral hyphae

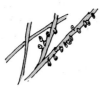

***Trichophyton rubrum***
Macronidia, rare small micronidia, with lateral
attachment to hyphae

***Malassesia furfur***
Short filaments and yeast cells
in skin scrapings

**Fig. 1.5** Morphology of some common dermatophytes.

or pressure sore. These should probably be regarded as secondary colonisers unless there is substantial clinical evidence of systemic or locally spreading infection.

**Note especially:**
- *Erysipelothrix rhusiopathiae* in butchers and fishmongers.
- *Corynebacterium diphtheriae* in people returning from Russia and the Indian subcontinent.
- *Haemophilus influenzae* as a cause of facial cellulitis in children.
- *Pasteurella multocida*, haemolytic streptococci, and mixed anaerobes in animal bites.

## Timesaving

- If the patient's condition justifies it, get the referring clinician to bring the specimen to the laboratory in person so that, if microscopy results are likely to have an impact on immediate clinical management, they can then be passed on in person.
- Where available, capillary gas–liquid chromatography can be used to demonstrate the presence of anaerobes in pus specimens.
- A metronidazole disk should be placed on one of the anaerobically incubated agar plates to give an early indication of the presence of obligate anaerobes.
- An ultraviolet lamp can be used to help confirm the presence of some slow-growing fastidious species such as *Prevotella melaninogenica*.
- If significant pathogens are isolated from a good quality specimen, preliminary culture results should be communicated to the requesting clinician as soon as they have been validated; if necessary, verbally.
- The written report should not have to wait for results of prolonged anaerobic incubation, or discretionary culture procedures for unusual soft tissue pathogens.

## Therapeutic issues

Sick patients with worsening constitutional symptoms or deteriorating local tissues need close attention. They may benefit more from surgical measures than from antibiotic therapy, but you need to ensure that the correct presumptive therapy is being given by the right route — usually i.v. In suspected myonecrosis, high dose i.v. benzyl penicillin should be given and, in suspected necrotising fasciitis, the treatment of choice is i.v. benzyl penicillin and clindamycin in combination (take care to avoid antibiotic associated colitis, though this is probably less common with clindamycin than once thought).

Topical antibiotics should be avoided. Their use has been clearly shown to often cause local sensitivity reactions and the rapid development of antibiotic resistance. If patients require antibiotic treatment for soft tissue infection, they will usually require at least an oral agent to ensure adequate levels of antibiotic in deeper infected tissues. Topical antiseptics in patients with burns represent an exceptional case in which specific antiseptic agents such as silver sulphadiazine have a special place. The use of steroid-containing creams should be avoided unless under the supervision of a dermatologist, in order to prevent an exacerbation of infective process.

Application of dressings to a skin defect is an important protection for exposed underlying tissues against secondary infection. Care should be taken in choice of dressing material to avoid: blocking the drainage of pus along a line of least resistance, overgrowth of potential pathogens under an occlusive dressing, and further damage due to shearing and tearing forces. A nurse with specialist training in wound care may be available to advise ward staff on dressings.

Providone iodine is commonly used as a topical antiseptic, but should not be applied to large areas of inflammation because of absorption and potential systemic toxicity. It may also have an antiphagocytic effect. Hypochlorite solutions are known to provoke superficial necrosis in some patients, dilute locally produced anti-infective factors and in the case of 'Eusol' have little disinfectant effect, while leaving a wet surface for subsequent growth of hospital bacteria such as *Pseudomonas aeruginosa*.

## Treatment of specific infections

- Actinomycosis requires 4–8 weeks penicillin therapy.
- Cutaneous anthrax: needs i.v. penicillin and anthrax antitoxin.
- Erysipeloid: give a penicillin or tetracycline, if no spontaneous remission.
- I.v. cannula-related: best results occur if cannula is removed.
- Pseudomonas may respond to removal of occlusion, drying and topical antiseptic.
- *S. pyogenes*: penicillin may need supplementing with flucloxacillin for staphylococcal coinfection.

## Prevention

Deep soft tissue infections, whilst dramatic in many respects, do not usually represent an infection hazard to other patients. Crusting, scaling, vesicular and exudative lesions, on the other hand, may present a substantial infection hazard. Exudate containing *S. aureus* or *S. pyogenes* and acute varicella-zoster lesions require additional control measures to prevent spread by contact or in dust particles. Hand hygiene measures for attending hospital staff, and a dressing covering the lesion should reduce the risk of cross infection. Cleaning, topical disinfectants and standard dressings will help prevent transmission from postoperative wounds even before the results of cultures are known.

The most important aspect of preventing infection of burned surfaces is meticulous hand hygiene by attending staff and application of topical antiseptics according to an agreed protocol. Cubicles do little to prevent infection in less severe burns, but may help staff practise good infection control. Burns patients in a general surgical ward should always be nursed in a single-bedded sideward.

## Follow-up

Results on any soft tissue specimen from a normally sterile site should be followed up by the microbiologist, especially if the problem was not drawn to the microbiologist's attention when first recognised by ward staff. It is also worth checking up on any patients whose wound swab was accompanied by a blood culture or whose clinical details suggest systemic infection.

Unexpected antibiotic resistance or slow growing soft tissue pathogens may provide a further opportunity to check the patient's response to therapy. Infections caused by 'alert' organisms such as *Streptococcus pyogenes* must also be followed up for infection control purposes, to check that control measures have been implemented and, if necessary, to introduce new measures.

# URINARY TRACT INFECTIONS

Urine specimens contribute a major proportion of the workload of a general diagnostic laboratory. Many will be normal or contain only contaminating organisms; and many of those patients with a significant microscopy or culture result will respond to a very brief course of oral antibiotic treatment. Consequently, the microbiology of urinary tract infection has an image problem. Too often it is regarded as 'routine', and quality suffers as a result.

## Troubleshooting

- If there is any doubt as to the significance of an isolate from a urine specimen, it may be resolved by requesting a further specimen (single isolate; 1st MSU = 80%, 2nd = 90%, 3rd = 100% confidence).
- Dipslide specimens may arrive from an out-of-the-way source. These should not be inoculated by micturition directly onto the agar paddle which makes identification of isolates difficult, and quantification of both bacteria and leukocytes impossible.
- Many MSU specimens come from patients with a very low probability of urinary tract infection. Some groups such as antenatal clinic attenders can be screened by urine dipstick test for nitrate reductase and leukocyte esterase. Gin-clear specimens that are negative for both are very unlikely to be positive on culture.
- The most common therapeutic errors in presumptive treatment of urinary tract infection-associated septicaemia are to leave the patient on oral antibiotics, and to continue with agents that are only really suited to uncomplicated cystitis.

## Specimen collection

As members of the commensal flora are also potential urinary pathogens, great care must be taken to avoid contamination during collection of a urine specimen. Particular problems occur when collecting specimens from female patients, paediatric urine bags, urinary catheters, ileal bladders and from patients with suspected renal tuberculosis.

*Females* Begin with a careful clean of external genitalia using plain soap and sterile gauze, separate labia with one hand, pass the first few drops of urine into the toilet, then direct urine flow into a sterile specimen container. Discard the last few drops of urine.

*Urine catheter* Drain contents of plastic tubing into a collection bag, disinfect specimen collection port, allow port to dry and further urine to collect in tubing, sample with sterile syringe and transfer to sterile specimen container.

*Elderly, incontinent* Males can have a condom device and bag applied after careful disinfection of the glans. Female patients are a problem and may require a 'clean catch' specimen collected while under supervision on the commode.

*Ileal bladder* The stoma should be thoroughly disinfected before passing a sterile catheter.

*Renal tuberculosis* The first urine of the day should be collected after careful cleaning of the external genitalia, to prevent contamination with commensal mycobacteria. Early morning specimens should be repeated on two further days; 24 h urine collections are unsuitable.

*N. gonorrhoeae* **or chlamydia culture** Unlike conventional MSUs, these should be the first 5–10 ml passed and need to be processed immediately.

*Schistosomiasis* To diagnose *Schistosoma haematobium* infection a urine specimen should be collected between 11 am and 5 pm after vigorous exercise.

*Paediatric bag urine* These specimens should be discouraged.

*Leptospirosis* Darkfield microscopy of urine is insensitive and prone to false positive results when performed by inexperienced staff. Culture usually takes too long to affect treatment choices.

## Specimen transport
Urine specimens deteriorate quickly. They should be cultured within 60 minutes. If this is not possible they should either be refrigerated at 4°C or passed into a borate urine container to give a final 1.8% w/v borate concentration.

## Specimen processing

### Microscopy
The preferred method uses an inverted light microscope to count the cells per high powered field in a microtitre well. Each microscope must be individually calibrated to allow conversion from cells/h.p.f. to cells/mm³. Wells should be inoculated with uncentrifuged urine by automatic pipette, according to a specimen template. Some laboratories use a microscope slide and coverslip method that is more prone to inaccuracy.

Urine leukocyte count can be increased by low urine flow and menstruation, and reduced by *Proteus* sp. infection or specimen collection in the early stages of urinary tract infection.

Causes of sterile pyuria include:

- prior antibiotic therapy
- tuberculosis
- urinary tract tumour
- urinary tract foreign body.

In suspected *S. haematobium* infection there should be a history of travel, and exposure to water. If a suitable specimen has been received (see above) centrifuge and examine the deposit for characteristic ova containing miracidia (Fig. 1.6).

There are rarely enough acid fast bacilli in the urine of patients with renal tuberculosis to produce a positive stain even after centrifugation, and false positive results can be caused by commensal mycobacteria.

### Culture
Cysteine lactose electrolyte-deficient (CLED) agar is commonly used as a single culture medium for urine specimens. Use a half plate per specimen.

 **The calibrated loop should be dipped vertically into the top of the hand-mixed specimen, and removed vertically without touching the side of the container.**

### Additional procedures
These are required in the following situations:

- Sterile pyuria: test for antibiotic substances in urine.
- Urethritis: culture for *N. gonorrhoeae* and chlamydias.
- Mycobacteria: culture of spun deposit, treated either with $H_2SO_4$ or N-acetyl-cysteine, on Lowenstein–Jensen.
- Suprapubic aspirate or ureteric urine: culture on blood anaerobically.
- If yeasts are seen on Gram stain: culture on Sabouraud's agar or similar.
- Viral infections (e.g. CMV) post-transplantation: neutralise acidic specimens with 7.5% $NaHCO_3$ and filter sterilise via 200 nm membrane; inoculate cell culture line.

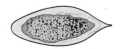

Terminal spine, 110–170 μm

**Fig. 1.6** Microscopic appearance of *Schistosoma haematobium*.

## Interpretation

No more than 10% cultures should have counts between $10^2$ and $10^4$ cfu/ml. If more than 10%, the quality of specimen collection is poor.

 The Kass criteria ($\geq 10^5$ cfu/ml in two fresh, carefully collected midstream urine specimens is highly predictive of bladder bacteriuria) apply only to women with cystitis, i.e. some patients will have infection with counts < $10^4$/ml.

Other situations where lower counts should be considered as evidence of infection especially if pure growth and pyuria present, include:

- staphylococci isolated
- pyelonephritis
- suprapubic or ureteric specimen
- recurrent cystitis
- enuresis.

Mixed cultures pose difficulties with interpretation unless one organism clearly predominates over all others. It is poor practice to request sensitivity testing on all bacteria isolated since the most common reason for mixed growth is contamination by perineal flora. If possible, request a further specimen taken under optimal collection conditions.

### Antibiotic sensitivities

Urine specimens with leukocytes and bacteria visible at microscopy can be put up on sensitivity agar on the same day as the primary culture plate to save time issuing the final report. However, this approach leads to loss of control over the inoculum density on the sensitivity plate, and is also prone to contamination by minority species.

While up to 8 antibiotics may be routinely tested against all urine isolates, only rarely will all 8 results be needed by the requesting clinician. Record all results but report selectively, where possible giving a choice of two or three agents suitable for treatment according to the clinical details given. It is helpful to divide your range of agents tested into first, second and third line agents for cystitis, pyelonephritis and urinary tract infection in pregnancy, and invasive infection with septicaemia. [Examples of each would be: nitrofurantoin, ampicillin and gentamicin, respectively.]

Antibiotics are unlikely to eradicate bacteriuria in the presence of a longterm indwelling urinary catheter but, if the patient has a fever or other features of severe infection, guidance on the choice of injectable antibiotics will be required.

## Follow-up

All specimens from patients with a fever or loin pain should be checked for a corresponding blood culture and culture results drawn to the attention of the medical staff in case antibiotic therapy needs modifying. Urinary tract infection-associated septicaemia usually responds rapidly to intravenous antibiotic treatment.

# IN THE LABORATORY

## BACTERIOLOGY

### IMPORTANT BACTERIAL SPECIES

### GRAM POSITIVE

*Actinomyces*
Facultative anaerobic, branching, Gram positive bacillus, catalase negative (except *A. viseosus*), produces acetic, succinic and lactic acids, but no propionic acid, metronidazole R.

*Bacillus*
Aerobic, sporeforming, Gram positive bacilli, usually forming large, spreading colonies on solid media. Most *Bacillus* spp. are not human pathogens. Two exceptions to this are:

● *B. cereus*: haemolytic, slightly green, motile, penicillin R
● *B. anthracis*: typical capsule, penicillin S, lysis with β-phage, nonmotile/nonhaemolytic.

*Clostridium*
Anaerobic, sporeforming, Gram positive bacillus (may stain Gram negative in later phase of growth) catalase-negative; oxidase negative; spores produced under anaerobic conditions.

*Corynebacterium*
Variably-shaped Gram positive bacilli, catalase positive; complex taxonomy currently under review.

*Enterococcus*
Facultative anaerobic, Gram positive cocci, in pairs or short chains, catalase negative, bile-aesculin/PYR/LAP all positive, NaCl (6.5%) tolerant and vancomycin S, may be streptococcal polysaccharide group D positive.

*Erysipelothrix*
Non-sporeforming Gram positive bacillus, catalase negative, nonmotile, $H_2S$ positive and (in TSI)/lactose positive, penicillin S, vancomycin R.

*Gardnerella*
Gram variable coccobacillus, facultative anaerobe, catalase negative, β-haemolytic on human blood agar, β-glycosidase/hippurate/starch all positive.

### Leuconostoc
Facultative anaerobe, Gram positive coccobacilli in pairs or chains; facultative anaerobe, catalase negative, LAP and PYR negative, vancomycin R.

### Listeria
Facultative anaerobe, short, non-spore-forming Gram positive bacilli, catalase positive and oxidase negative; acid from glucose, aesculin hydrolysis, tumbling motility at 22°C.

### Pediococcus
Facultative anaerobe, Gram positive cocci in clusters, quartets or pairs; catalase negative, LAP positive, PYR negative, vancomycin R.

### Peptostreptococcus
Strictly anaerobic, Gram positive coccus, colonies not pigmented black, vancomycin S.

### Propionibacterium
Anaerobic, Gram positive bacillus, catalase negative; reduces nitrate, produces acetic, succinic and propionic acids, metronidazole R.

### Staphylococcus
Gram positive cocci, in clusters. facultative anaerobes. catalase positive:

- *S. aureus*: coagulase, protein A, DNAase all positive.
- *S. epidermidis*/other coagulase-negative staphylococci: coagulase/protein A/DNAase negative; Novobiocin R = *S. saprophyticus*.

### Streptococcus
Gram positive cocci, in chains of variable length, catalase negative:

*β-haemolytic* Clearing around colonies on blood agar; i.d. by latex agglutination of capsular polysaccharide.

- Group A: *S. pyogenes* and some '*S. milleri*' isolates, *S. pyogenes* PYR positive, *S. milleri* PYR negative/VP positive.
- Group B: *S. agalactiae*, also CAMP test positive but may be non-haemolytic.
- Group C: includes *S. equi; equisimilis* and *zooepidemicus*; some '*S. milleri*' isolates.
- Group F: some '*S. milleri*' isolates.
- Group G: some '*S. milleri*' isolates, others.

*α-and non-haemolytic*

- *S. pneumoniae*: optichin S and bile salt soluble.
- *S. bovis*: bile-aesculin positive, optichin negative, bile salt negative.
- Viridans group: all three tests negative.
- nutritionally variant streptococci: PYR positive, satellitism.

## GRAM NEGATIVE

### Acinetobacter
Gram negative bacillus, oxidase negative, nonfermenter, DNAse negative, nonmotile, non-pigmented, nitrate negative.

### Aeromonas
Facultative anaerobic, Gram negative bacillus, motile, oxidase positive, variable growth on TCBS, growth on nutrient agar without NaCl, but not on NA with 6% NaCl vibriostatic agent 0/129 R, usually indole positive and gas from glucose.

### Bacteroides
Anaerobic, Gram negative bacillus, nonpigmented, vancomycin and kanamycin R.

### Bordetella
Aerobic, Gram negative coccobacillus, asaccharolytic, most common sp. (*B. pertussis*) does not grow on conventional non-selective agars; requires Bordet–Gengou or similar, agglutination test positive.

### Branhamella (redesignated Moraxella) catarrhalis
Gram negative diplococcus, oxidase positive, grows on nutrient agar at 37°, no acid from glucose, maltose, sucrose or maltose, DNAase positive, nitrate positive.

### Brucella
Aerobic, Gram negative coccobacillus, catalase and oxidase positive, glucose and lactose nonfermenters, nonhaemolytic, positive agglutination test (anti-smooth Brucella serum).

### Burkholderia
Aerobic, Gram negative bacillus, oxidase positive (apart from *B. gladioli* and *B. mallei*), growth on MAC, no growth on Cetrimide (apart from *B. cepacia*); other tests vary according to spp.

### Campylobacter
Microaerophilic, Gram negative bacillus, most spp. grow on selective solid media containing antibiotics; not all spp. grow at the most commonly used incubation temperature (42°C). Non-selective media at 37°C for unusual *Campylobacter* spp. in sterile fluids.

### Capnocytophaga
Capnophilic, facultative anaerobic, slender Gram negative bacilli with tapered ends, gliding motility, usually aminoglycoside resistant:
— DF-1 group: catalase, oxidase, ADH all negative
— DF-2 group: catalase, oxidase, ADH all positive (*C. canimorsus* and DF-2 like; *C. cynodegmi*).

### Cardiobacterium hominis
Capnophilic, pleomorphic Gram negative bacillus (may be coryneform or form rosettes), catalase negative, oxidase and indole positive, glucose and maltose positive, lactose and xylose negative.

### Citrobacter
Facultative anaerobic, Gram negative bacillus, oxidase negative, more common spp. usually lactose fermentation, motile, citrate positive, ONPG positive, gas from glucose, mannitol positive, urease, VP, LDC all negative.

### Eikenella corrodens
Capnophilic, facultative anaerobic, Gram negative bacillus, pitting colonies on agar, oxidase positive; catalase negative, nonmotile, nonsaccharolytic, ODC and LDC positive, but ADH, urease, gelatin all negative.

### Enterobacter
Facultative anaerobic, Gram negative bacillus, variable lactose fermentation, motile, ONPG positive, gas from glucose, VP, citrate, ODC all positive, urease and indole negative.

### Escherichia coli
Facultative anaerobic, Gram negative bacillus, oxidase negative, usually lactose fermenter; indole positive, ONPG and LDC positive, gas from glucose, motile; urease, VP, citrate and, PPA negative (D-sorbitol positive, apart from almost all *E. coli* O157:H7).

### Flavobacterium (redesignated Chryseobacterium)
Gram negative bacillus, oxidase and catalase positive, pigmented colonies, nonmotile, nonfermenter, hydrolyses gelatin, polymyxin B R resistant, acid from maltose, no growth on MAC, indole positive.

### Fusobacterium
Anaerobic, Gram negative bacillus with tapered ends, indole positive. *F. necrophorum* and *F. mortiferum* very pleomorphic.

### Haemophilus
Small Gram negative coccobacillus, usually with fastidious growth requirements, and growth enhanced by a humid atmosphere with 5% $CO_2$, satellite growth next to *S. aureus* streak or XV disk on primary isolation medium. Porphyrin test from δ-aminolaevulinic acid.

### Helicobacter
Microaerophilic, Gram negative (often curved or spiral) bacillus, motile, catalase, oxidase and $H_2S$ positive on TSI, no growth at 25 or 42°C. *H. pylori*: rapid urease positive.

### Kingella
Facultative anaerobic, Gram negative coccobacillus, oxidase positive, usually catalase negative, and acidifies only glucose, nitrate positive, nonmotile.

### Klebsiella
Facultative anaerobic, Gram negative bacillus, oxidase negative, usually lactose fermenter, often mucoid colonies, ONPG, VP, citrate and urease positive, gas from glucose, mannitol/sucrose/salicin all positive, nonmotile, VP and indole negative, some spp. indole positive.

### Legionella
Aerobic, slender Gram negative bacillus, requiring L-cysteine for growth, which is enhanced by iron salts and $CO_2$, asaccharolytic, most spp. catalase and oxidase positive, motile.

### Moraxella
Gram negative coccobacillus, often in pairs, oxidase and catalase positive, asaccharolytic, most spp. urease negative, no growth on MAC, penicillin S.

### Neisseria gonorrhoeae
$CO_2$-enriched growth, Gram negative diplococcus, oxidase positive, acid from glucose, but not from maltose, sucrose or lactose, DNAase negative.

### Neisseria meningitidis
$CO_2$-enriched growth, Gram negative diplococcus, oxidase positive, acid from glucose and maltose, but not from sucrose or lactose, DNAase negative.

### Pasteurella
Facultative anaerobic, Gram negative coccobacillus, catalase, oxidase, indole and sucrose positive; usually ODC positive, no growth on MAC, penicillin S.

### Prevotella
Anaerobic, Gram negative bacillus, either black pigmented colonies or red fluoresence under UV light, vancomycin and kanamycin R.

### Proteus
Facultative anaerobic, Gram negative bacillus, non-lactose fermenter; motile, ONPG negative, gas from glucose, $H_2S$ and urease positive, LDC negative; some spp. indole positive, tendency to swarm on agar surface.

### Pseudomonas
Aerobic, Gram negative bacillus, oxidase positive, motile, usually grows on MAC (nonfermenter), more common spp. pigmented, produce acid from glucose (oxidative). *Ps. aeruginosa* will grow at 42°C.

### Salmonella
Facultative anaerobic, Gram negative bacillus, non-lactose fermenter; ONPG negative, motile; $H_2S$, LDC and mannitol positive, indole, urease and VP negative.

### Shigella
Facultative anaerobic, Gram negative bacillus, nonmotile, usually non-lactose fermentation (apart from *S. sonnei*), ONPG negative (apart from *S. sonnei* and some *S. dysenteriae*); VP, citrate, urease, $H_2S$ and LDC negative.

### Stenotrophomonas (formerly Xanthomonas)
Gram negative bacillus, oxidase negative, aesculin and DNAase positive, hydrolyses gelatin, LDC positive, Colistin S.

### Vibrio
Facultative anaerobic, Gram negative (often curved) bacillus, oxidase positive, growth on TCBS. *V. cholerae* produces yellow colonies; other yellow Vibrio spp., *V. alginolyticus*, *V. fluvialis*, *V. furnissii*, *V. metschnikovii*; rest are green. Vibriostatic test (0/129) positive, string test positive, motile, more common spp. LDC and ODC positive.

### Yersinia
Facultative anaerobic, Gram negative bacillus, nonlactose fermenter … usually ONPG positive, methyl red, urea and nitrate positive, no gas from glucose, VP, citrate and $H_2S$ negative, nonmotile.

## ACID FAST

### Mycobacterium
Aerobic, non-spore-forming, strongly acid-fast bacillus, with slow to very slow rates of growth. Results of preliminary identification tests for more commonly encountered species are given below. Gene probes are available for identification of *M. tuberculosis*, *bovis*, *avium complex*, *kansasii* and *gordonae*.

**M. tuberculosis** Slow growing acid fast bacillus, non-pigmented, optimum = 37°C, rough colonies, niacin and nitrate positive.

**M. avium complex** Slow growing acid fast bacillus, non-pigmented, optimum = 37°C, smooth and thin or rough, colonies niacin and nitrate negative.

**M. kansasii** Slow growing acid fast bacillus, photochromogen, optimum = 37°C, intermediate to rough colonies, niacin/nitrate both negative.

**M. malmoense** Slow growing acid fast bacillus, nonpigmented, optimum = 37°C, smooth colonies, niacin/nitrate, both negative.

**M. ulcerans** Slow growing acid fast bacillus, nonpigmented, optimum = 30°C, rough colonies, niacin/nitrate both negative.

*M. marinum* Moderately fast growing acid fast bacillus, photochromogen, optimum = 30°C, smooth to intermediate, rough colonies, niacin/nitrate both negative.

*M. chelonae* Rapid growing acid fast bacillus, nonpigmented, optimum = 28°C, smooth or rough colonies, growth on MAC, niacin positive or negative, nitrate negative.

*M. fortuitum* Rapid growing acid fast bacillus, nonpigmented, optimum = 28°C, smooth or rough colonies, with filamentous projections, growth on MAC, niacin positive or negative, nitrate positive.

### Nocardia

Aerobic, moderately acid-fast, branching, filamentous Gram positive bacilli, catalase positive; usually lysosyme resistant, dry, rugose colonies after prolonged incubation on nonselective media.

## RECENT NAME CHANGES

It is essential to use the correct name when reporting a pathogen isolated from a clinical specimen. From time to time the officially recognised name of a given genus or species may be changed to reflect changes in internationally agreed taxonomy. In recent years developments in molecular microbiology have challenged the phenotypic basis for naming many medically important species. Listed below in Table 2.1 are some of the more important changes in bacterial nomenclature.

**TABLE 2.1 Important recent name changes**

| Previous name | New name |
| --- | --- |
| **Gram positives** | |
| Arachnia propionica | Propionibacterium propionica |
| Corynebacterium haemolyticum | Arcanobacterium haemolyticum |
| CDC group JK corynebacteria | Corynebacterium jeikeium |
| Corynebacterium pyogenes | Actinomyces pyogenes |
| Peptococcus spp. | Peptostreptococcus, most spp. |
| Streptococcus faecalis | Enterococcus faecalis |
| Streptococcus faecium | Enterococcus faecium |
| **Gram negatives** | |
| Achromobacter xylosoxidans | Alcaligines xylosoxidans subsp. xylosoxidans |
| Acinetobacter calcoaceticus var anitratus, most | Acinetobacter baumanii |
| Bacteroides gingivalis | Porphyromonas gingivalis |
| Bacteroides gracilis | Campylobacter gracilis |

**TABLE 2.1   Important recent name changes (cont'd)**

| | |
|---|---|
| Bacteroides melaninogenicus | Prevotella melaninogenica |
| Bacteroides salivosus | Porphyromonas salivosa |
| Campylobacter butzleri | Arcobacter butzleri |
| Campylobacter cinaedi | Helicobacter cinaedi |
| Campylobacter laridis | Campylobacter lari |
| Campylobacter pylori/pyloridis | Helicobacter pylori |
| Citrobacter diversus | Citrobacter koserii |
| Erwinia herbicola | Pantoea herbicola |
| Flavobacterium meningosepticum | Chryseobacterium meningosepticum |
| Haemophilus aegyptius | Haemophilus influenzae biogroup aegyptius |
| Moraxella catarrhalis | Branhamella catarrhalis |
| Moraxella kingii | Kingella kingii |
| Pasteurella maltocida, some | Pasteurella canis |
| Pasteurella ureae | Actinobacillus ureae |
| Proteus morganii | Morganella morganii |
| Pseudomonas cepacia | Burkholderia cepacia |
| Pseudomonas diminuta | Brevundimonas diminuta |
| Pseudomonas gladioli | Burkholderia gladioli |
| Pseudomonas paucimobilis | Burkholderia pickettii |
| Pseudomonas pickettii | Burkholderia pseudomallei |
| Pseudomonas pseudomallei | Sphingomonas paucimobilis |
| Pseudomonas putrifasciens | Shewanella putrifasciens |
| Rochalimea henselae | Bartonella henselae |
| Rochalimea quintana | Bartonella quintana |
| TWAR strain chlamydia | Chlamydia pneumoniae |
| Wolinella recta | Campylobacter recta |
| Xanthomonas maltophilia | Stenotrophomonas maltophilia |

## ANTIBIOTIC SUSCEPTIBILITY TESTING

Many different methods of detecting antibiotic resistance are used. The most commonly used in routine diagnostic practice are forms of disk diffusion test; the Stokes (comparative) (Table 2.2) and Kirby–Bauer (Table 2.3) methods. Both methods aim to identify acquired antibiotic resistance that might result in treatment failure.

Although results can be reported as sensitive, intermediate or resistant, the 'intermediate' category is of little help to clinicians and should be avoided on final laboratory reports if at all possible.

**TABLE 2.2   Antibiotic disks for Stokes comparative method**

| | |
|---|---|
| **Staphylococci** | |
| Penicillin | 2 iu |
| Methicillin | 5 µg |
| Cephradine/Cephalexin | 30 µg |
| Erythromycin | 5 µg |
| Fucidic acid | 10 µg |
| Rifampicin | 5 µg |
| Chloramphenicol | 10 µg |
| Vancomycin | 30 µg |
| **Streptococci** | |
| Penicillin | 0.25 iu |
| Ampicillin | 10 µg (enterococci) |
| Cephradine/Cephalexin | 30 µg |
| Erythromycin | 5 µg |
| Chloramphenicol | 10 µg |
| Vancomycin | 30 µg |
| **Haemophilus** | |
| Ampicillin | 2 µg |
| Erythromycin | 5 µg |
| Chloramphenicol | 10 µg |
| Cefotaxime | 10 µg |
| **Neisseria gonorrhoeae** | |
| Penicillin | 0.01 iu |
| Penicillin | 0.25 iu |
| Penicillin | 1 iu |
| Spectinomycin | 100 µg |
| Tetracycline | 10 µg |
| Ciprofloxacin | 1 µg |
| **Enterobacteriaceae, non-urinary** | |
| Ampicillin | 10 µg |
| Cephradine/Cephalexin | 30 µg |
| Gentamicin | 10 µg |
| Cefotaxime/Ceftriaxone | 10 µg |
| Ciprofloxacin | 1 µg |
| **Urinary isolates** | |
| Trimethoprim | 2.5 µg |
| Nitrofurantoin | 50 µg |
| Nalidixic acid | 30 µg |
| Ampicillin | 10 µg |
| Cephradine/Cephalexin | 30 µg |
| Gentamicin | 10 µg |
| Ciprofloxacin | 1 µg |

**TABLE 2.2  Antibiotic disks for Stokes comparative method (cont'd)**

*Pseudomonas, miscellaneous hospital Gram negative bacilli*

| | |
|---|---|
| Gentamicin | 10 μg |
| Amikacin | 30 μg |
| Piperacillin | 30 μg |
| Ciprofloxacin | 1 μg |
| Imipenem | 10 μg |

**TABLE 2.3  Antibiotic disk inhibition zone sizes for the Kirby–Bauer method**

| | Susceptible (mm) | Resistant (mm) |
|---|---|---|
| **Staphylococci** | | |
| Penicillin G | ≥ 29 | ≤ 28 |
| Methicillin | ≥ 14 | ≤ 9 |
| Cefazolin | ≥ 18 | ≤ 14 |
| Erythromycin | ≥ 23 | ≤ 13 |
| Rifampicin | ≥ 20 | ≤ 16 |
| Chloramphenicol | ≥ 18 | ≤ 12 |
| Vancomycin | ≥ 12 | ≤ 9 |
| **Streptococci** | | |
| Penicillin | ≥ 28 | ≤ 19 (not *S. pneumoniae*) |
| Ampicillin | ≥ 17 | ≤ 16 (enterococci) |
| | ≥ 30 | ≤ 21 (not *S. pneumoniae*) |
| Erythromycin | ≥ 23 | ≤ 13 |
| Chloramphenicol | ≥ 18 | ≤ 12 |
| Vancomycin | ≥ 17 | ≤ 14 (enterococci) |
| | ≥ 12 | ≤ 9 |
| **Enterobacteriaceae, non-urinary** | | |
| Ampicillin | ≥ 17 | ≤ 13 |
| Cefaclor | ≥ 18 | ≤ 14 |
| Gentamicin | ≥ 15 | ≤ 12 |
| Cefotaxime | ≥ 23 | ≤ 14 |
| Ciprofloxacin | ≥ 21 | ≤ 15 |
| **Urinary isolates** | | |
| Trimethoprim | ≥ 16 | < 10 |
| Nitrofurantoin | ≥ 17 | < 14 |
| Nalidixic acid | ≥ 19 | < 13 |
| Gentamicin | ≥ 15 | ≤ 12 |
| Ciprofloxacin | ≥ 21 | ≤ 15 |

**TABLE 2.3  Antibiotic disk inhibition zone sizes for the Kirby–Bauer method (cont'd)**

| Pseudomonas, miscellaneous hospital Gram negative bacilli | | |
| --- | --- | --- |
| Gentamicin | ≥ 15 | ≤ 12 |
| Amikacin | ≥ 17 | ≤ 14 |
| Piperacillin | ≥ 18 | ≤ 17 (*Pseudomonas*) |
| | ≥ 21 | ≤ 17 (other spp.) |
| Ciprofloxacin | ≥ 21 | ≤ 15 |
| Imipenem | ≥ 16 | ≤ 13 |

NB These zone sizes only apply if the susceptibility test method used follows the recommendations of the National Council for Clinical Laboratory Standards for media, inoculation, antibiotic disks and incubation [NCCLS M2-A5 and M7-A3].

Note Zone sizes between susceptible and resistant NCCLS thresholds are regarded as 'intermediate'.

The Comité de l'Antibiogram de la Société Française de Microbiologie has recommended different zone interpretation criteria in Statement 1996 CA–SFM. These criteria and the corresponding susceptibility testing methods can be found in a supplement to Clinical Microbiology and Infection 1996 2(supp.): S1–49.

## Reporting sensitivity results

When reporting sensitivity test results remember that you are giving guidance to the clinician on the antibiotics you think suitable or unsuitable choices for treatment. Avoid using the 'intermediate' category if at all possible, and do not report bug–drug combinations that appear sensitive in the laboratory but make unsuitable choices of treatment, e.g. nitrofurantoin 'sensitive' *Proteus* sp., or gentamicin 'sensitive' *Salmonella typhi*. It is better to avoid reporting these combinations altogether, but some laboratories choose to report them always as resistant irrespective of laboratory result.

It is helpful to the requesting clinician to restrict the choice of antibiotics to a few that would be suitable for use in that particular clinical setting, e.g. first line agents for uncomplicated cystitis. However, you will need to report a much wider choice if the patient is seriously ill. A reduced choice of agents due to multiple antibiotic resistance in a clinically significant isolate should prompt additional sensitivity testing.

## Specific problems in sensitivity testing

Interpretive standards are difficult to set for fastidious bacteria (i.e. *Haemophilus influenzae*, *S. pneumoniae*, *Neisseria* spp., fastidious anaerobic spp.) and fungi. Some laboratories where the Kirby–Bauer method is used overcome the problem by using the Stokes comparative method for fastidious bacteria.

Staphylococci may produce intermediate or even 'sensitive' zones of penicillin inhibition despite having β-lactamase. These should be reported resistant if the edge of the zone is heaped up or ragged.

An oxacillin 1 μg disk is preferred to a methicillin disk by some laboratories because of slower deterioration in storage. Sensitivity to either should be tested on Mueller–Hinton agar incubated at 30°C or half-strength salt-containing Mueller–Hinton agar at 35°C.

β-lactamases produced by *Klebsiella* spp. ensure that clinical isolates are functionally resistant to ampicillin even if the zone diameter suggests they are sensitive. For a similar reason, if Enterobacteriaceae are resistant to ampicillin, they are also resistant to piperacillin, irrespective of piperacillin zone size.

Some β-lactamases produced by Gram negative bacilli may not be detected by conventional disk diffusion testing. As this type of resistance is becoming more common in hospital isolates of Enterobacteriaceae and is often associated with aminoglycoside modifying enzymes, aminoglycoside resistant hospital isolates should be tested using the double-disk inhibition method in which a cephalosporin disk such as cefotaxime is placed close to an amoxycillin-clavulanic acid disk to look for combined inhibition where the diffusion zones overlap.

Antibiotic disks deteriorate quickly, particularly in the case of some β-lactam agents exposed to moisture. When not in use, disks should be stored in a dessicator and refrigerated. The dessicator should be brought to room temperature to avoid condensation at the start of each work period.

## EPIDEMIOLOGICAL METHODS IN COMMON USE

The diagnostic laboratory has a role to play in confirming an apparent time–space cluster as an outbreak, whether in hospital or in the surrounding community. The provisional identification of a primary source and means of transmission will usually be based on:

- the identity of the microbial pathogen
- the type of infection
- time/place/person data.

A growing list of laboratory methods has been applied in epidemiological investigations; however the information they provide cannot better the quality of specimen and data collection.

Laboratory methods can be extremely helpful in either confirming or refuting an epidemiological hypothesis, but only rarely contribute much to the initial containment of an outbreak.

Laboratory typing methods aim to subdivide members of a given species (see Table 2.4). To be of practical use the chosen method should be quick and easy to perform, and produce a large number of reproducible subtypes. This does not always apply to molecular methods!

TABLE 2.4    Laboratory typing methods

| Organism | Method |
| --- | --- |
| Acinetobacter baumannii | Serotyping, PCR |
| Candida albicans | REA, PFGE |
| Enterobacteriaceae | Plasmid typing, REA, PCR, PFGE |
| Enterococci | Ribotyping, PGFE |
| Klebsiella spp. | Serotyping, REA, PCR, PFGE |
| Mycobacterium tuberculosis | Southern blot/IS6110, PFGE |
| Pseudomonas aeruginosa | Pyocine, PCR, PFGE |
| Salmonella spp. | Serotyping, phage, plasmid, RFLP |
| Staphylococcus aureus | Phage, plasmid, PCR, PFGE |
| Streptococcus pneumoniae | Capsular serotyping |

## ROUGH GUIDE TO MOLECULAR EPIDEMIOLOGY

### PLASMID TYPING

Gel electrophoresis of extrachromosomal DNA may allow differentiation of different types during an outbreak. However, a single plasmid band difference is not necessarily significant since plasmids may be lost from clinical isolates during storage, or there may be open and closed variants of the same plasmid with differing electrophoretic mobilities. A more reliable method is to use restriction endonuclease enzymes (REA) (e.g. BamI or HinDIII) to cut plasmid DNA into shorter lengths before electrophoresis.

### Restriction endonuclease analysis (REA)

The use of restriction endonuclease enzymes to cut plasmid or chromosomal DNA into shorter lengths before electrophoresis produces a large number of bands or restriction fragments. The differences in band pattern due to varying restriction fragment lengths permits differentiation of types, but so many bands may be generated that this becomes subjective.

### Polymerase chain reaction (PCR)

PCR has been used to amplify gene sequences in a variety of typing methods. Commonly used methods include arbitrarily-primed PCR or randomly-amplified PCR (low stringency reaction conditions to ensure multiple bands on electrophoresis), and repetitive extragenic palindromic sequence analysis (cryptic DNA sequences of variable length). RAPD is easier to perform but less reproducible than REP sequence typing. Both methods can be applied across a range of bacterial species. Some PCR-based methods have been adapted to typing of specific genera.

## Pulsed field gel electrophoresis (PFGE)

PFGE allows separation of large DNA fragments into relatively few bands and is suited to analysis of chromosomal DNA cut with low frequency restriction endonucleases. Results are highly reproducible but the method is technically demanding and may take several days to perform.

## Southern blotting

In a Southern blot, bacterial DNA separated by gel electrophoresis after digestion by restriction endonuclease action is then transferred ('blotted') onto nitrocellulose membrane. A probe specific to a homologous DNA sequence is then applied to the membrane.

## Ribotyping

In ribotyping, the Southern blot method is used to demonstrate DNA sequences associated with the ribosomal operon. The method produces highly reproducible results for a wide range of baterial genera but requires a high degree of skill and equipping.

Molecular evidence that two isolates belong to idential clones is not conclusive evidence that transmission has taken place. All that typing methods can do is indicate the relatedness of isolates; not the sequence, duration or direction of transmission. It follows that evidence for transmission from source A to patient B must be based on classic epidemiological principles. The role of a molecular method is to support an epidemiological investigation by adding weight to or refuting a working hypothesis.

# VIROLOGY

## AIDS AND HIV

### DIAGNOSIS

A diagnosis of AIDS is usually considered as a result of an indicator infection or other marker pathology. Confirmation of CDC stage requires detailed analysis of T cell subsets by flow cytometry and HIV serum markers. Cytometry should demonstrate an abnormally low CD 4+ cell count and/or a reduced CD 4+ percentage of T cells, when compared against age-specific normal ranges. In young children, opportunist infections may occur despite a normal CD4+ count, so HIV status must be assessed. Antibodies to p24, gp41, 120 and 160 can be detected by ELISA, but all positives should be confirmed by repeat test, if necessary, using a second ELISA method. HIV serology in newborns and young children is problematic. Where available, PCR detection of viral RNA may be useful, but assessment normally relies on mothers' serological results and repeating tests for HIV serum markers at intervals up to 18 months of age.

### Prognosis

The median interval between onset of seropositivity and AIDS is around 10 years, with a further 2 years to death. Antiretroviral therapy can prolong both the time to development of AIDS and the AIDS–death interval. Combinations of antiretroviral drugs have been shown to be more effective than a single agent, and for maximum effect should now consist of two reverse transcriptase inhibitors and a protease inhibitor.

### Legal and ethical considerations

Tests for HIV serum markers should not be performed without counselling the patient and obtaining their consent. In critically ill patients it is occasionally necessary to assess HIV status without prior consent. When this has to be done it is the attending clinician's decision, and arrangements must be made for future counselling.

Healthcare workers who become HIV seropositive may, in rare circumstances, represent a risk to patients and colleagues. If they choose to continue working, they should be placed under proper medical supervision. This is best done via the staff or occupational health department who can maintain professional confidentiality. Staff engaged in procedures likely to involve contact between their blood and the patients, tissues (e.g. surgeons) may have to be redeployed.

## HEPATITIS MARKERS

Hepatitis A and E only cause acute infection; while B, C and D may cause chronic disease.

### Hepatitis A: anti-HAV IgM, anti-HAV IgG
Single serum specimen for confirmation of acute HAV infection by IgM, or single serum specimen for assessment of HAV immune status by IgG.

### Hepatitis B: HBsAg/HBcAbIgM
HBV DNA or HBeAg positive early in symptomatic period. Surface antigen positive shortly before onset of symptom and anti-core (HBcAbIgM) positive around onset. Anti-core IgM (HBcAbIgM) indicates recent acute infection, while anti HBcIgG indicates past infection. Anti HBs is used for evidence of immunity following immunisation. In chronic hepatitis B carrier state, HBe antigen positive indicates high risk and HBe antigen negative a correspondingly low risk.

### Hepatitis C: anti HCV
Positives should be confirmed with second test method, and where available by PCR for viral RNA; negatives should be followed up with repeat test after 3–6 min if chronic disease.

### Hepatitis D: (fulminant or exacerbation of hepatitis B)
False negative results are common; test therefore is unreliable.

### Hepatitis E: anti-HEV
The test is available in some reference centres but this disease is uncommon in developed countries.

# PARASITOLOGY

## LEISHMANIA ENDEMIC AREAS

The geographical distribution of members of the genus *Leishmania* — cause of cutaneous, mucocutaneous and visceral leishmaniasis — is complex and depends on exposure to infected sandflies (*Lutzomia* spp. in the Americas and *Phlebotomus* spp. elsewhere). Different forms of the disease are distributed as follows:

*Visceral leishmaniasis*

- Mediterranean littoral.
- Pockets in the Middle East.
- Horn of Africa.

**TABLE 2.5   Differential characteristics of microfilariae**

|                  | 1  W. bancrofti                              | 2 B. malayi                           | 3 L. loa                               |
|------------------|----------------------------------------------|---------------------------------------|----------------------------------------|
| Length (μm)      | 200–300                                      | 220–250                               | 250–300                                |
| Diameter (μm)    | 8                                            | 6                                     | 8                                      |
| Sheath           | Present (stains lightly with Giemsa)         | Present (stains deeply with Giemsa)   | Present (almost colourless with Giemsa)|
| Body curves      | Regular, smoothly curved                     | Irregular, twisted                    | Irregular, twisted                     |
| Cephalic space   | Small                                        | Large                                 | Large                                  |
| Body nuclei      | Coarse, well separated                       | Coarse, tend to overlap               | Coarse, tend to overlap                |
| Tail end         | No nuclei, pointed tip                        | 2 widely-spaced nuclei, blunt tip     | Nuclei present, rounded tip            |
| Location in host | Blood, hydrocele fluid Chylous urine         | Blood                                 | Blood                                  |
| Periodicity      | Nocturnal subperiodic                        | Nocturnal subperiodic                 | Diurnal                                |

Reproduced with permission: Zaman V and Loh S. Handbook of Medical Parasitology, 1978, Churchill Livingstone, Edinburgh UK.

- India (eastern coasts), Bangladesh, Burma.
- Pockets in mainland China.
- Parts of South America (*L. chagasi*).

*'Old World' cutaneous leishmaniasis*

- Mediterranean littoral.
- Pockets in northern half of sub-Saharan Africa.

*'New World' mucocutaneous leishmaniasis*

- Central America and north-eastern parts of South America.

## Microfilaria morphology (→ Table 2.5)

| 4 O. volvulus | 5 M. perstans | 6 M. streptocerca | 7 M. ozzardi |
|---|---|---|---|
| 250–300 | 150–200 | 180–240 | 150–200 |
| 8 | 4 | 5 | 4 |
| Absent | Absent | Absent | Absent |
| Regular, slightly twisted | Regular, often forms loops | Tail usually curved | Regular, slightly twisted |
| Large and bulbous | Large | Large | Large |
| Coarse, mostly separated | Medium sized, tend to overlap | Fine, mostly separated | Fine, mostly separated |
| No nuclei, rounded tip | Nuclei present, rounded tip | Nuclei present, curved tip | No nuclei, pointed tip |
| Skin | Blood | Skin | Blood and skin |
| None | None | None | None |

## Serodiagnosis of parasitic infections

The prolonged incubation period of many parasite infections means that demonstration of a rising antibody titre may not be possible. Moreover, a measurable antibody response to a given parasite epitope may not necessarily be associated with significant morbidity. Nevertheless, serodiagnostic techniques have some applications in clinical parasitology, as shown in Table 2.6.

**TABLE 2.6   Serodiagnosis of parasitic infections**

| Serological tests | Indications |
| --- | --- |
| **Useful** | |
| Toxoplasmosis | congenital, recent infection, IgM |
| Cysticercosis | may be negative in CNS infection |
| Echinococcosis | more positive in hepatic disease<br>ELISA or HIA, confirmed by arc 5 IEP |
| Amoebiasis | IHA or ELISA positive in all hepatic and<br>70% intestinal infections |
| Toxocariasis | ELISA, false positive possible in some endophthalmitis |
| Filariasis | in blood film negative patients |
| Strongyloidiasis | ELISA usually positive |
| **Occasionally useful** | |
| Leishmaniasis | high level ELISA or IFA titre may indicate recent/active<br>visceral infection |
| Malaria | screening for infected blood donor |
| Schistosomiasis | positive result should prompt search for eggs |

# ENTOMOLOGY

## DISEASES TRANSMITTED BY ARTHROPOD VECTORS

Some of the most common infections worldwide are transmitted by arthropods. The more important vectors and the common infections spread by these vectors are summarised in Table 2.7.

Key morphological features of the more common arthropod vectors of disease are shown in Figures 2.1–2.5. These diagrams can be annotated to show features of locally important vector species.

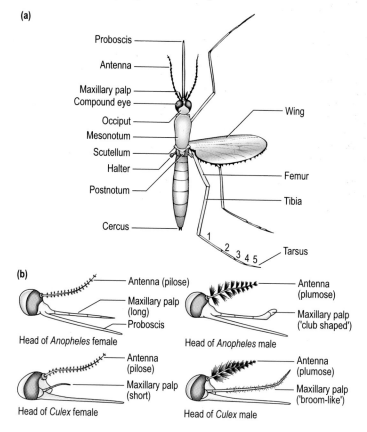

**Fig. 2.1** Adult mosquito. (a) General features. (b) Head parts of Anopheles and Culex mosquitoes. (Redrawn with permission for Zaman V, Keong L 1989 *Handbook of medical parasitology* Churchill Livingstone, Edinburgh)

**TABLE 2.7   Disease vectors and common associated infections**

| Vectors | Disease |
| --- | --- |
| Mosquitoes | Malaria |
| | Filariasis |
| | Arbovirus infections |
| Sandflies | Leishmaniasis |
| | Papatasi fever |
| | Bartonellosis |
| Tsetse flies | African trypanosomiasis |
| Blackflies | Onchocerciasis |
| Tabanid flies | Loa loa |
| Fleas | Plague |
| | Murine typhus |
| Lice | Epidemic typhus |
| | Epidemic relapsing fever |
| Reduviid bugs | Chagas' disease |

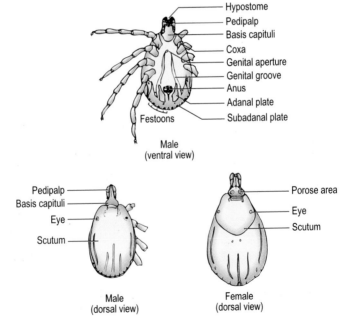

Male
(ventral view)

Male
(dorsal view)

Female
(dorsal view)

**Fig. 2.2** Morphological features of hard ticks. (Redrawn with permission for Zaman V, Keong L 1989 *Handbook of medical parasitology* Churchill Livingstone, Edinburgh)

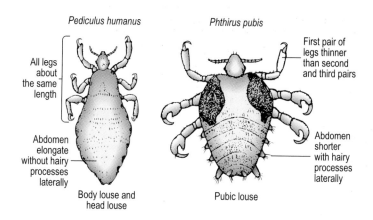

*Pediculus humanus*

All legs about the same length

Abdomen elongate without hairy processes laterally

Body louse and head louse

*Phthirus pubis*

First pair of legs thinner than second and third pairs

Abdomen shorter with hairy processes laterally

Pubic louse

**Fig. 2.3** Lice commonly found on humans. (Redrawn with permission for Zaman V, Keong L 1989 *Handbook of medical parasitology* Churchill Livingstone, Edinburgh)

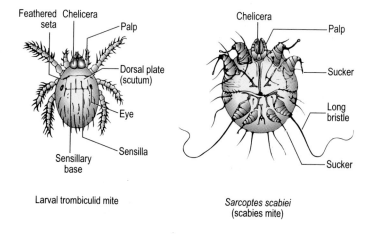

Feathered seta   Chelicera — Palp

Dorsal plate (scutum)

Eye

Sensilla

Sensillary base

Larval trombiculid mite

Chelicera — Palp

Sucker

Long bristle

Sucker

*Sarcoptes scabiei* (scabies mite)

**Fig. 2.4** Two common varieties of mite. (Redrawn with permission for Zaman V, Keong L 1989 *Handbook of medical parasitology* Churchill Livingstone, Edinburgh)

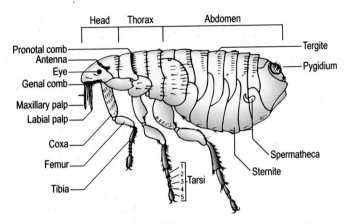

**Fig. 2.5** Generalised adult flea. (Redrawn with permission for Zaman V, Keong L 1989 *Handbook of medical parasitology* Churchill Livingstone, Edinburgh)

# GENERAL LABORATORY ISSUES

## ACCREDITATION

Diagnostic laboratories in the UK and many other countries benchmark their work by formal accreditation. There are different bodies for different types of laboratory and different countries. Consequently, there are major differences in the way laboratories can gain formal accreditation.

The principal accrediting body in the UK is the Clinical Pathology Accreditation (CPA), an agency set up as a result of collaboration between the Royal College of Pathologists and other interested organisations. CPA accreditation is not compulsory to date, but has been sought by most hospital laboratories in response to competition from the private sector.

By applying for accreditation, a laboratory effectively submits its activities to objective, external quality control. Accreditation itself does little more than set the seal on claims to have reached an externally assessed standard. But the preparation for a visit by the accrediting body's inspectors may start a standard-improving process in a diagnostic laboratory. However, the benefits of accreditation will only be passed to requesting clinicians and their patients if the improvement process is sustained. Most accrediting agencies require recertification of participants after a defined period, and may also expect a mid-cycle report, e.g. on improvements made at the request of inspectors. There is little point in working for accreditation if there is no intention to continue in the scheme after the first certification.

Some schemes (e.g. ISO) concentrate on written documentation of laboratory processes. While it might appear to be easier to obtain certification through documentation alone, such schemes are unlikely to encourage improvements in pre and post analytical determinants of laboratory results. As microbiology services are not medically-led in many US hospitals, the scheme operated by the College of American Pathologists may place microbiology at a disadvantage against other branches of laboratory medicine. The infection control component of medical microbiology is particularly prone to be overlooked, unless a specific request is made for review during inspection.

CPA uses the following main headings:

- organisation & administration
- staffing & direction
- facilities & equipment
- policies & processes
- staff development & education
- evaluation.

## INFORMATION MANAGEMENT

In information terms, the diagnostic laboratory responds to a request by processing an accompanying clinical specimen and subsequently issues a report. The speed and accuracy of that report is the principal determinant of the laboratory's clinical efficiency (see Reporting and Turnaround Times, below).

Copies of laboratory reports must be kept for future reference. How you choose to store your copies is a managerial decision but if it does not allow easy access this will soon become apparent. Whatever the method you must be able to find a copy quickly yourself, but the information should be protected against loss through theft, fire and computer failure. There should also be an 'audit trail' that allows the work performed to be followed through from specimen receipt to report dispatch and attributed to specific members of staff.

Clerical and secretarial staff will handle all of the laboratory's requests and reports (input and output) at least once. They may also be the first voice heard by anyone calling for information, and consequently the first to handle criticism of the laboratory's service. Calls from impatient colleagues should be handled promptly and courteously by the most senior member of staff at hand.

### Hazards of paper-free reporting

The paper-free laboratory will experience greater difficulty amending reports, especially if several investigations are being run in parallel. The timing of print runs may drive the entire laboratory timetable. Electronic reports rarely allow much room for explanations of complex results and may encourage excessive data reduction at the transcription level. Direct electronic transfer to wards can also push the laboratory further away from clinical practice.

Avoid direct or implied criticism of the laboratory's information management; it will only reduce your own credibility.

Finally, information stored in electronic format must comply with data protection legislation.

## LOST SPECIMENS

- Few, if any, specimens go missing in a well-run laboratory; more often specimens are lost before arriving in the lab.
- It should be possible to track a specimen through the entire course of processing, even if the original specimen has long since been discarded.

There are all sorts of reasons why you may want to find a specimen quickly. Most often it will be to answer a telephone enquiry while the caller is still on the line. The following usually works:

1. Ask the caller for the patient's name, unit, the specimen type, and the time of specimen collection. If it was sent out of hours, establish whether or not it was an urgent specimen.
2. Check that the specimen has been received by the lab:
   - Is there an entry in the booking-in ledger?
   - Has it been logged into the lab computer?
   - If it hasn't yet arrived, check with nursing staff on the ward/unit:
     - Was the specimen collected?
     - Did it leave the ward?
     - What transport arrangements were made.
3. Obtain the lab accession number.
4. Ask the MLSO in charge of handling the relevant specimen type if they have the specimen.
5. If this doesn't work, get the caller's contact number and promise to call back later. Then:
   - ask a secretary to track the request forward
   - ask a senior MLSO to track the specimen back.
6. Remember to return the call.

## OUT-OF-HOURS MICROSCOPY

- The microscope used for diagnostic work out-of-hours is often the most heavily used in the department.
- It will not always be left in optimal condition by the previous user.
- The controls and objective lenses may be different to your usual microscope.

### General problems

- Difficulty getting a sharp focus under oil immersion: try cleaning the immersion lens with xylene. If that does not work, try recentering the substage condenser.
- Eyes tiring after prolonged sessions peering down the microscope: check there is a blue filter below the substage condenser.
- Always remember to clean immersion oil off immediately after use. It could be you using the microscope next.

## Wet films

### Lost the plane of view?

1. Go back to the edge of the coverslip, refocus, and move it back into view.
2. Sometimes suspended material settles at the fluid/air interface along one of the 4 edges, so it may be worth following the edge.
3. Failing that, mark the slide with wax crayon or felt-tip next to the coverslip, focus and move back over the coverslip.

## Gram stain

### Cannot find anything at all under high power?

- Is it a very light smear?
- Did you forget to heat fix before staining?
- Is the smear on the underside of the slide?
- Are you viewing the right end of the slide?
- Are you in the correct focal plane?

### Too heavy to make out any detail?

- Decolourisation is more difficult to get right. Go to edge of smear where material should be thinner.

### Gram variable organisms
These can be due to:

- easily decolourised species (e.g. *Clostridia*)
- semiviable bacteria (e.g. *streptococci*)
- underdecolourised bacteria.

Scan several adjacent fields under oil to see if effect is uniform. (Stain deposit looks like Gram-positive cocci of variable diameter.)

## Zeihl–Neelsen (Z–N) stain

As very few bacilli may be present, you can only be sure that a smear is negative after:

- concentration by centrifugation, and
- examination either for 15 minutes or 50 high power fields.

This is rarely possible on-call, so negative smears and the respective specimen should be kept for repeat processing according to standard laboratory protocol during normal working hours.

A strong positive can often be detected quickly in an unconcentrated acid-fast smear by selecting a dense collection of neutrophils, and scanning over it using a × 40 objective. Even if positive at this magnification, the morphology of possible acid-fast bacilli should still be checked under the immersion lens.

Note the density of AFBs (+ to ++++), and the presence of beading and cords.

If an auramine-rhodamine method is used, remember that yeasts can produce fluorescing acid-fast bodies.

### Staining for Nocardia or Actinomycetes?

Remember that these genera are less acid-fast and require a weaker acid in the decolourisation step.

### Spore stain (Albert's)

This is a modified version of the Z–N. If requested for exudate, blister fluid or tissue from a patient with suspected gas gangrene/clostridial myonecrosis. Remember that Clostridia rarely produce spores during the acute stage of severe disease.

## Toluidine blue for PCP

This is a simple stain suitable as an on-call alternative to monoclonal antibody or calcofluor white for *Pneumocystis carinii* in bronchoalveolar lavage fluids. Expectorated sputum is usually unsuitable for examination.

Cysts (reddish blue–purple) are best found in flecks of mucoid material.

## OUT-OF-HOURS SPECIMENS

Arrangements for dealing with out-of-hours specimens in your laboratory will depend on out-of-hours staffing, specimen transport and the location of temporary storage facilities. These arrangements will be written down somewhere, and should be available to all laboratory users.

### Specimens that will arrive out-of-hours

*Urgent specimen* The result is likely to have immediate impact on patient management; arrange immediate transport/priority processing.

*Unrepeatable specimen* These are dangerous, difficult or costly to repeat.

- Immediate transport or processing required.
- Adequate storage facilities on ward/unit.

### Specimens that should arrive but do not

*No specimen* Patient has either died, got better, been transferred to another doctor/ward, or the working diagnosis has changed.

### Specimen in transit

- Left at collection point — bedside, operating theatre, or ward treatment room.

- Wrong storage — ward fridge, holding incubator for BCs.
- In system as routine/non-urgent.

*Specimen in laboratory*

- Awaiting booking-in/processing.
- Held up in haematology, biochemistry, histopathology.
- Packed with non-urgent specimens.
- Arrived with no label/request form.

## Specimens that should not arrive

Easily repeated, non-urgent specimens and specimens that cannot be processed or stored out of hours. Note circumstances and request repeat during working hours.

## Unsafe specimens

Contact sending unit to request repeat, or advise a delay in results. Only handle the original if you have adequate safety equipment, and a colleague present to answer the phone and assist with other urgent work.

## Specimen transport

This should be for no more than 2 h at ambient room temperature, and less than 15 min if fastidious bacteria are expected. Specialised transport media are required for *Neisserias, Chlamydias*, and viruses. Most easily cultivated anaerobic bacteria will survive short transport periods without the need for a transport medium. CSF should never be refrigerated prior to bacterial culture.

## Specimen storage

If immediate processing is not possible/required, storage at ambient room temperature is usually satisfactory up to 24 h maximum. Faeces, urines, sputum or viral transport medium should be stored at 4°C.

## Rejected specimens

Specimens arriving out-of-hours without a request form or label, after prolonged transport, in leaking containers, or in duplicate, may be unsuitable for processing. If there is a genuine concern that they will produce unreliable or frankly misleading results, they can be discarded, providing you:

- note circumstances
- contact sending unit and inform
- give reason for rejection on report form.

You may also want to hold specimen for 24 h as a further back-up.

## QUALITY ASSURANCE AND CONTROL

The laboratory will only have an impact on clinical practice if its work is reliable. Each time a given specimen is processed, the requesting clinician should have the same level of confidence in the result, unless notified of a change in laboratory practice. However, in many respects, microbiology is a qualitative science and so, to ensure consistently high standards, regular internal checks must be performed. This is internal quality control, and should be directly supervised by a senior member of the scientific staff in conjunction with a senior medical microbiologist.

Key issues in quality control include regular sterility checks and assessment of the growth support properties of in-house media, positive, negative and calibration controls, operating ranges of incubators, policing of reagent shelf-life, compliance with agreed protocols, and the upkeep of an error/remedial action logbook.

Various external bodies support internal quality control activities by running external quality assurance (EQA) schemes in which mock-up specimens are sent to the participating laboratory for processing. Results are returned to the organisers for marking. A summary of all participants' results is then sent out as a stimulus to correct major discrepancies from the intended result. Clearly, schemes such as NEQAS (UK) and CAP (USA) rely on QA specimens being processed alongside routine specimens of the same type. Handing QA specimens over to senior staff (or worse, to another laboratory) for processing defeats the object of the exercise. If the laboratory is unable to assure a reliable result for a given specimen, specimens of that type should be sent on to a more suitable laboratory.

Do not discard QA specimens as soon as processing has been completed. They often contain pathogens less commonly seen in smaller diagnostic laboratories and therefore represent a useful source of teaching material for junior staff.

## REPORTING AND INTERPRETATION

- The report is the laboratory's principal means of outgoing communication with its users.
- Each report will be incorporated into the patient's medical record, and may have a significant impact on clinical management decisions.

### Laboratory worksheets

All procedures undertaken on clinical specimens must be recorded so that specimen processing can be followed retrospectively for problem-solving, quality assurance and audit purposes. The referring clinician does not require any of this detail, whether in abbreviated form or otherwise. However, it is vital that a record is kept of what was done; in particular: any potentially significant observation, the basis for any procedural decisions taken, and any deviation from standard laboratory protocol.

There must be some record on the worksheet of who has performed the tests, and when they were done. Any senior staff who have validated observations or results should add their signature against the date.

### Preliminary or interim reports

Your laboratory should be prepared to provide a statement of initial observations on the same day as initial results are obtained. This is particularly important for urgent specimens whose results may have an immediate impact on patient management, and for specimens whose processing is likely to significantly exceed the normal turnaround time.

### Final reports

You should seek to state the laboratory's observations in a relatively simple, standardised form. If the result requires interpretation, be prepared to add a brief comment. A succinct statement in neat handwriting is more likely to be read than a computer-generated general comment. Where relevant, reference ranges should be given as a guide to interpretation. Only clinically relevant pathogens and antibiotic susceptibility results should be reported.

All results should be subject to medical authorisation before releasing the final report on the final day of specimen processing, though high-volume negative results may be delegated to senior members of laboratory staff. Extra copies or amended reports may be required in some cases. You must ensure that all reports, whether verbal or written, are treated as confidential out of respect for the patient's privacy.

### Computerised/direct reporting

Computerisation has sped up aspects of the reporting process and made laboratory results more accessible but remember the following:

- The volume of reports generated is not a function of their accuracy or clinical relevance.
- Only data that has been entered into the computer can be analysed with it.
- A comprehensive computer system will dictate lab workflow patterns and speed.
- Direct reporting to the ward removes one of the most useful interfaces with clinical staff.

## SAFETY IN THE LABORATORY

## LEGAL BACKGROUND

Employer and employee both have responsibility for the maintenance of a safe working place. This extends beyond biological hazards to include chemical, electrical, radioactive and fire hazards. However, diagnostic microbiology laboratories are unique in the scale and variety of potential biohazards they may harbour. The remainder of this section will concentrate on biological hazards in the diagnostic laboratory. Biological agents capable of causing disease have been classified under EC Directive (93/88/EEC).

Lab safety is now governed in many countries by legislation. In the UK the general background is provided by Health and Safety at Work (HSW) Acts. More recently, safety conditions have been tightened up considerably. In particular, control measures for the containment of biological agents are now mandatory for any laboratories where these are handled (see CoSHH 1994 and EC Directive 90/679/EEC). Safety considerations are interwoven into requirements for laboratory accreditation, and standards should meet those required by current legislation.

## Categories of biological hazard (hazard groups)

These are summarised in Table 2.8. Most medically important bacteria are in hazard group 2; none are in group 4 which contains only viruses. Important examples from groups 3 and 4 are given below:

**TABLE 2.8   Categories of biological hazard**

| Group | Human disease | Hazard to employees | Community spread | Prophylaxis or treatment |
|-------|---------------|---------------------|------------------|--------------------------|
| 1 | unlikely | none | none | |
| 2 | possible | possible | unlikely | available |
| 3 | possible | serious | possible | available |
| 4 | severe | serious | likely | none |

*Hazard group 3*

- Bacteria: *B. anthracis, Brucella* spp., *B. pseudomallei* and *mallei, C. psittaci, C. burnettii, M. tuberculosis* and other mycobacteria; *Rickettsia* spp., *Salmonella typhi* and *paratyphi*.
- Fungi: *Blastomyces* spp., *Coccidiodiomyces* sp., *Histoplasma capsulatum, Paracoccidioides brasiliensis, Penicillium marneffii*.
- Parasites: *Echinococcus, Leishmania, Naegleria, Plasmodium falciparum, Taenia solium, Trypanosoma cruzi* and *rhodesiense*.
- Prion agents: CJD, GSS, kuru.
- Viruses: LCM, hantavirus, dengue virus, yellow fever, hepatitis B, C, and D, HIV, HTLVI and II, rabies.

*Hazard group 4*   Lassa, Ebola, Marburg, Congo-Crimean haemorrhagic fever viruses. Further details can be found in: Advisory Committee on Dangerous Pathogens 1995. Categorisation of biological agents capable of causing infection, 4th edn. HMSO, HSE Books, Sudbury, UK.

## Risk assessment

In addition to the hazard group rating of a given microorganism, the following factors should be taken into account when assessing biological risk:

- virulence
- transmissibility
- route or routes of infection
- quantity handled
- type of work
- extent of dissemination
- steps needed to prevent, control or contain.

## Higher level biocontainment

The level of biological containment normally corresponds to the hazard group of the pathogen(s) you are working with. Most laboratory work you undertake will be at biocontainment level 2. Details of safe working practice for this and all other levels can be found in the ACDP booklet referred to above. If the clinical specimens or other material you process are likely to contain pathogens from hazard groups 2 and 3, you should perform your work in a biocontainment level 3 laboratory.

*A level 3 lab* is a specially designated, separate room. It will be restricted to authorised access. It should seal completely in case radical decontamination is required. There will be negative pressure ventilation, the exhaust being vented via a double HEPA filter system. Inside, the lab should have an exhaust-ventilated biological safety cabinet, arrangements for storing organisms, and for safe disposal of infected waste. Finally, there will be a washbasin in the room, or its anteroom, and there should be an observation window in the door.

## Biological safety cabinets

A variety of biological safety cabinets (BSCs) are found in diagnostic microbiology laboratories. They will only protect the user if they are used properly and maintained carefully. Laminar flow cabinets and fume cupboards are not designed to provide protection against biological agents.

*Class I* This is an open front cabinet that draws in air at the front and expels it from a separate filtered exhaust. It is suitable for all microbial pathogens up to and including hazard group 3. Airflow should be checked by anemometer reading weekly if in daily use. Readings should be taken at the four corners and the centre of the opening and the mean calculated. The range should be between 0.7 m/sec and 1.0 m/sec, with no reading varying by more than 20% of mean. Integral airflow indicators are prone to inaccuracy and should only be used as a guide.

*Class II* This is an open front cabinet that recirculates some filtered air, while drawing in replacement air via the front. Some protection is offered but maintenance is difficult and it is unsuitable for pathogens in hazard groups 3 and 4.

*Class III* This cabinet provides a complete physical barrier between operator and pathogens. All exhaust is filtered. It is suitable for hazard group 4 pathogens.

Maintenance of all BSCs should only be performed by service engineers with appropriate training and experience. Further details can be found in: Advisory Committee on Dangerous Pathogens 1995. Categorisation of biological agents capable of causing infection, 4th edn. HMSO, HSE Books, Sudbury, UK.

## TURNAROUND TIMES

Turnaround times are a measurable function of laboratory performance and are now required in diagnostic laboratory protocols. There are three components: transport, laboratory processing, and report generation. The lab has little control over transport times, but should complete processing of most specimens within 72 h.

In practice, the referring clinician is most interested in an overall turnaround time, i.e. from specimen collection to final report. Answers to enquiries about how long before a result is ready must be based on a detailed knowledge of specimen processing and report generation in your own laboratory. The following standards are general guidelines:

### Laboratory turnaround

*Blood culture* Preliminary results should be reported immediately by the fastest reliable means, and an interim report should be made on all cultures within 48 h.

*CSF* Preliminary results should be reported immediately by the fastest reliable means.

*Faeces* Highly variable.

*Sputa* Final report by 3 days, and any atypical pathogens should be reported within 2 months.

*Urines* Majority should be reported within 24 h and all routine specimens within 48 h.

*Wound exudate, swabs* Highly variable.

*Virology* Variable, since high cost of reagents dictates batch processing.

Based on: S. Mehtar (ed) 1994 Guidelines for standards in laboratory practice in medical microbiology. Association of Medical Microbiologists, No 3.

# ANTIBIOTIC USE

## ANTIFUNGAL THERAPY

### Candidaemia

Around 25% cases have a negative blood culture; there is a mortality rate of 40%. Treatment options are as follows:

- If **cannula associated** and there is no evidence of dissemination, remove cannula and repeat blood culture. Give 400 mg fluconazole i.v. on 1st day, then 200 mg daily and continue up to 4 weeks max. Amphotericin is an alternative.
- For **other patients** including immune compromised, disseminated infections need more aggressive therapy. Give an i.v. amphotericin 1 mg test dose in 50 ml 5% dextrose over 2 h; then increase over 7 d to 0.6–0.8 mg/kg each day.
- **Severely ill** patients need to increase to maximum dose over 24 h and may benefit from i.v. flucytosine 200 mg/kg in 4 doses each day.
- **Candida endocarditis** will not respond to antifungal agents alone. Early surgical intervention is needed. Continue therapy for at least 4 more weeks.

### Cryptococcal meningitis

Treatment of choice is i.v. amphotericin and flucytosine. In patients who are not HIV positive, fluconazole has been used as an alternative.

### Rhinocerebral mucormycosis

This requires high dose i.v. amphotericin and radical excision.

### USING I.V. AMPHOTERICIN

When given i.v. amphotericin can cause a wide variety of toxic and other adverse effects including: fever, rigors, backache, headache, vomiting, phlebitis, anaemia and hypokalaemia. In many cases it will cause some degree of renal damage. Nevertheless, amphotericin remains the agent of choice for several deep or systemic fungal infections. The risk of toxic reactions and other adverse effects can be reduced by:

- giving a 1 mg test dose in 50 ml 5% dextrose over 2 h
- steady increase to maximum dose over 7 d
- using 50 mg hydrocortisone with the infusion
- replacing infusion with 5% dextrose if signs of reaction.

Monitor temperature, blood pressure, urea and electrolytes (particularly magnesium) frequently during amphotericin therapy. If flucytosine is being used as well, remember to monitor levels to guide dosage (serum flucytosine should not be allowed to rise above 80 mg/l).

 Any immunocompromised patient with systemic fungal infection will have a better chance of response to antifungal therapy if the underlying disease process can be reversed.

# CONTRAINDICATIONS FOR ORAL ANTIBIOTICS

**TABLE 3.1  Contraindications for oral antibiotics**

| *All agents:* | *History of hypersensitivity* |
|---|---|
| Albendazole | Pregnancy |
| Cephalosporins | Acute porphyria |
| Chloramphenicol | Pregnancy, breast feeding, porphyria |
| Clindamycin | Diarrhoea |
| Erythromycin | Avoid estolate in liver disease |
| Ethambutol | Optic neuritis, poor vision, young children |
| Foscarnet | Pregnancy, breast feeding |
| Griseofulvin | Pregnancy, SLE, porphyria, liver failure |
| Halofantrine | Pregnancy, breast feeding, sycope attacks, prolongation of QT interval |
| Isoniazid | Drug induced liver disease |
| Mefloquine | Pregnancy, 1st trimester |
| Nitrofurantoin | Infants < 3 months, G6PD deficiency, porphyria |
| Pyrazinamide | Liver damage, porphyria |
| Quinine | Haemoglobinuria, optic neuritis |
| Ribavirin | Pregnancy |
| Rifampicin | Jaundice, porphyria |
| Sodium stibogluconate | Breast feeding, renal failure |
| Tetracyclines | Pregnancy, breast feeding, < 12 years old, renal failure, systemic lupus |
| Thiabendazole | Pregnancy, breast feeding |
| Trimethoprim | Pregnancy, neonates, blood dyscrasias, renal failure |
| Zidovudine | Neutropoenia, anaemia, hyperbilirubinaemia in newborns |

# INTRAVENOUS ANTIBIOTICS

## INTRAVENOUS DOSES

The doses listed below are for a 70 kg adult with normal renal and liver function.

 **Prior history of hypersensitivity is a contraindication. Penicillin hypersensitivity implies crossreactivity to all penicillins and possibly to cephalosporins.**

*Acyclovir* See page 2.

*Amphotericin* See pages 102–103.

*Ampicillin* 500 mg i.v. every 6 h.

*Aztreonam*

- Septicaemia: 1–2 g i.v. every 6–12 h.
- Severe UTl: 500–1000 mg every 12 h.

*Benzyl penicillin*

- 1.2 g i.v. every 6 h.
- 2.4 g i.v. every 4 h to start with for meningitis; 1.8–2.4 g 4-hourly for lobar pneumonia.

*Cefotaxime*

- Septicaemia: 1–2 g every 8 h i.v.
- Severe UTI: 1 g every 12 h i.v.
- Avoid in acute porphyria.

*Ceftriaxone*

- 1–2 g i.v. every 12 or 24 h; limited experience in septicaemia.
- Avoid in acute porphyria.
- Avoid in infants < 6 months (hepatorenal impairment).

*Cephradine*

- 500 mg–1 g every 6 h i.v. but avoid if also in use for prophylaxis.
- Avoid in acute porphyria.

*Chloramphenicol*

- 500 mg every 6 h i.v.; 50 mg/kg daily dose to maximum of 1 g daily.
- Dose-dependent marrow depression effect ceases on stopping therapy, goes in 2–3 weeks.
- Irreversible aplastic anaemia at 1 in 20 000.

*Ciprofloxacin*

- 500 mg every 12 h p.o. if tolerated.
- 400 mg for life-threatening infections.
- Stop therapy if tendon inflammation/damage.

*Erythromycin*

- 500 mg every 6 h i.v. 1 g every 6 h in legionnaires' disease.
- Avoid if possible in liver disease.

*Flucloxacillin* 1 g every 6 h i.v. 1–2 g every 6 h for bone/joint infections.

*Fluconazole* see under Antifungal therapy, above.

*Fusidic acid*

- 500 mg every 8 h i.v. by slow infusion.
- Avoid in severe liver disease.

*Gentamicin*

- If 70 kg adult and normal renal function, 120 mg leading dose and 100 mg 8-hourly thereafter.
- Dose depends on renal function, weight and previous serum levels.
- Avoid in pregnancy and myasthenia gravis.

*Meropenem*

- 500 mg every 8 h i.v. preferable to imipenem/cilastatin — lower epilepsy risk

*Metronidazole*

- 500 mg every 8 h i.v.
- Avoid in severe liver disease, and established neurological disease, particularly convulsive disorders.

*Penicillin*

- 1.2 g i.v. every 6–12 h.
- 2.4 g i.v. every 3 h to start with for meningitis; 1.8–2.4 g every 4 h for lobar pneumonia.

*Rifampicin*

- 1.2 g every 12 h p.o. if possible; i.v. by slow infusion.
- Avoid in jaundice and severe liver disease.

*Vancomycin*

- 500 mg–1 g every 12 h i.v. to start; subsequent dosage according to serum levels given by slow infusion.
- Rotate infusion sites.

## LIVER FAILURE AND ANTIBIOTICS

 Toxicity may be difficult to predict as the hepatic reserve is usually large. Liver function tests are a poor guide to metabolic activity.

### Avoid

The following should be avoided in liver failure:

- Chloramphenicol, due to higher risk of marrow suppression.
- Fusidic acid; reduce dose if use is absolutely necessary.
- Isoniazid; toxicity is more common.
- Pyrazinamide: toxicity more common.
- Rifampicin; if use essential, do not exceed 8 mg/kg daily.
- Tetracyclines; dose-related toxicity.

### Reduce dose

Reduce dose of the following in patients with liver failure:

- Ceftriaxone; monitor plasma concentration if hepatorenal failure.
- Clindamycin.
- Meropenem; monitor bilirubin and transaminase.
- Metronidazole; in severe disease.
- Terbinafine.

# NEUROSURGICAL PROPHYLAXIS

A recent working party report stated that clinical trial results suggest that antibiotic prophylaxis may be beneficial in clean neurosurgical procedures. Cephalosporins were the preferred choice; e.g. cephradine or cephazolin 1 g i.v. at induction followed by a further 500 mg for every three hours during prolonged procedures.

The same working party was unable to find convincing evidence that antibiotic prophylaxis prevented infection following basal skull fracture or in the presence of a dural tear / CSF leak, and noted the possible increased risk of infection with antibiotic resistant bacteria. They observed that the few recent trials fail to show a benefit in terms of reduced incidence of meningitis. (Ref: Brown EM 1993 Antibiotic prophylaxis in neurosurgery. Journal of Antimicrobial Chemotherapy 31 (Supp B): 49–63)

# PENICILLIN ALLERGY

## Emergency management

Features of acute anaphylaxis are: nausea, vomiting, pallor, tachycardia, severe dyspnoea, abdominal pain, rigors, loss of consciousness, with or without acute urticaria or angioneurotic oedema [mortality is~~ 10%].
Treatment is as follows:

1. 500–1000 µg adrenaline i.m. Repeat every 15 min until signs of improvement.
2. 10–20 mg chlorpheniramine (or alternative antihistamine) by slow i.v. injection after adrenaline. Repeat over next 24–48 h to prevent relapse.

## Late reactions

These occur around 7–10 days after antibiotic administration and resemble a serum sickness type of illness with fever, rash and polyarthralgia. They usually respond to withdrawal of antibiotic therapy.

## Assessing risk of hypersensitivity reaction

Concern about hypersensitivity reaction is the most common reason for avoiding use of penicillin antibiotics. Anaphylactic reactions occur at a rate of between 0.004% and 0.04% and happen less than 72 hours after starting treatment, sometimes within minutes.

There are problems assessing the risk of a hypersensitivity reaction by skin testing. Patch testing with benzyl penicillin can provoke an anaphylactic reaction. The less reactive artificial substitute, penicillyl-polylysine (PPL), can miss up to 3% reactors, especially those with an anaphylactic tendency. A second skin test reagent, suitable for detection of so-called minor determinants, can substantially reduce the risk of missing reactors when used in combination with PPL. However, this second reagent is not commercially available and is only used in a few major centres with a special interest. More recently, some centres have turned to lymphocyte transformation tests to assess risk of hypersensitivity reaction. Although skin tests may not be widely available they do show that around three-quarters of patients who think they are allergic to penicillin do not react at all.

Clearly, the only method of assessing risk in most centres is a carefully taken therapeutic history. Any previous mention of antibiotic allergy or reaction in the patient's record should be checked with the patient, and changes in the patient's account clearly documented in the record. Ampicillin rash appears to be most common (circa 10%, in infectious mononucleosis circa 90%) and in some cases may be a toxic, dose-related phenomenon. There is around 3–9% cross sensitivity with cephalosporins, which should also be asked for in all cases of suspected penicillin reaction.

# PREGNANCY AND ANTIBIOTICS

- **If possible, avoid use of all antibiotics during 1st trimester.**
- **Use only if benefits to mother outweigh risk to fetus.**

## Antibiotics not known to be harmful

These are:

- penicillins
- cephalosporins
- clindamycin.

## Antibiotics to avoid in pregnancy

- Aminoglycosides: monitor if use is essential.
- Chloramphenicol: risk of grey baby syndrome late in pregnancy.
- Colistin: risk of fetal toxicity.
- Dapsone: risk of neonatal haemolysis and methaemoglobinaemia.
- Fluconazole: manufacturer's advice.
- Flucytosine: teratogenic risk.
- Foscarnet: manufacturer's advice.
- Ganciclovir: teratogenic risk.
- Griseofulvin.
- Ketoconazole.
- Metronidazole: avoid high dose regimens.
- Nitrofurantoin: risk of neonatal haemolysis if close to term.
- Sulphonamides: risk of neonatal haemolysis and methaemoglobinaemia.
- Tetracyclines: risk of maternal hepatotoxicity at high dose; risk of dental discolouration.
- Tribavirin.

- **Specific antimalarial agents pose a threat to the fetus but maternal benefit usually exceeds fetal risk.**
- **Check risk of individual agents before use.**

# PRESUMPTIVE ANTIMICROBIAL CHEMOTHERAPY

You will only rarely be asked for advice on choosing antibiotics for an infection for which a definitive aetiological diagnosis has already been made. Recommendations for presumptive antibiotic therapy are, by definition, made without specific laboratory guidance. That does not mean that your advice will be less rational. See the relevant item in the clinical problems section for presumptive therapy of a specified syndrome.

## General principles

1. Try to establish a working diagnosis on the basis of existing information.
2. Review the most likely microbial pathogens.
3. Ensure that a serious attempt is made to obtain all the relevant diagnostic specimens, preferably before commencing therapy.
4. Check that there are no contraindications to any major groups of antimicrobial agents (e.g. known allergies or deteriorating renal function).
5. Recommend the smallest number of antimicrobial agents with the narrowest possible antimicrobial range for the most likely pathogens, according to local susceptibility results.
6. Review the patient's clinical progress and lab results at least once.

## Do not

- Forget alternative infectious and noninfectious conditions in the differential diagnosis.
- Try to 'cover' all possible pathogens with your antibiotic choice.

## Giving a second opinion

For many possible different reasons, you may have to add your opinion to an already complicated clinical picture. This may be an opportunity to rescue a deteriorating situation by contributing a distinctively different perspective. Remember that you have the advantage of hindsight, and that you are seeking a change in the clinical consensus. Moreover as a pathologist, you are an outsider whose opinion has been invited, but which can just as easily be ignored. General points to follow:

- Find out as much as you can about what has happened so far, and what has been done by your colleagues.
- Avoid open, personal criticism and value judgements about a colleague's professional practice.
- Attempt to understand why a given approach was taken.
- In the absence of specific clues, it is wise to make only one major antibiotic change at a time.

- If clinical improvement coincides with a new antibiotic, it may be possible to dispense with other agents that were started previously, even if the aetiology is not yet known.
- Review the patient's clinical progress and lab results at least once more.

# RENAL FAILURE AND ANTIBIOTICS

## Avoid if possible

- Chloramphenicol: in severe renal failure there is higher risk of dose-related marrow suppression.
- Mefloquine: avoid for prophylaxis in mild failure.
- Nalidixic acid: unsuitable for UTI in moderate failure.
- Nitrofurantoin: unsuitable for UTI in moderate failure.
- Povidone iodine: especially repeated application to mucosa/broken skin in severe failure.
- Proguanil: avoid for prophylaxis in severe failure.
- Tetracycline: avoid in mild failure.
- Vancomycin: avoid if possible in mild failure.

## Reduce dose

- Acyclovir: reduce dose in moderate/severe failure.
- Amoxycillin/ampicillin: reduce in severe failure.
- Aztreonam: reduce in moderate failure.
- Benzyl penicillin: in severe failure, maximum dose is 6 g per day.
- Cefotaxime: halve dose in severe failure.
- Ceftriaxone: reduce dose in severe failure.
- Cephradine: reduce dose in mild failure.
- Chloroquine: reduce dose in mild/moderate failure.
- Ciprofloxacin: halve dose in moderate failure.
- Clarithromycin: reduce dose in moderate failure.
- Erythromycin: maximum adult does is 1.5 g daily in severe failure.
- Ethambutol: reduce dose in mild failure.
- Fluconazole: reduce dose in mild failure.
- Flucytosine: reduce dose in mild failure.
- Foscarnet: reduce dose in mild failure.
- Isoniazid: maximum adult dose of 200 mg daily in severe failure.
- Meropenem: reduce dose in mild failure.
- Pentamidine: reduce dose in mild failure.
- Piperacillin: reduce dose in mild failure.
- Teicoplanin: reduce dose after 4 d in mild failure.
- Terbinafine: halve dose in mild failure.
- Trimethoprim: reduce dose in mild failure.

## POST-SPLENECTOMY PROPHYLAXIS

The risk of major infection following splenectomy is relatively low, but still represents a preventable cause of death. Risk is highest in children, particularly after spelenectomy for thalassaemia or lymphoma. The most common cause of infection is *Streptococcus pneumoniae*.

23-valent pneumococcal vaccine should be given 2 weeks before elective splenectomy, and immediately after traumatic splenectomy. As protective antibody levels decline, a booster should be given 3–6 years later. The Hib vaccine should be given to children not already vaccinated against *Haemophilus* infection, and in those less than 5 years old. Give daily prophylactic penicillin V for 2 years or until postvaccination seroconversion.

Advise patients of the importance of seeking early medical action in the event of infection. They should also be warned to avoid animal bites and scratches. (See Read RC, Finch RG 1994 Journal of Antimicrobial Chemotherapy 33: 4–6.)

# THERAPEUTIC DRUG MONITORING

- Some institutions have a policy of not performing antibiotic assays on body fluids out-of-hours.
- Antibiotic levels are only usually measured for agents with a significant risk of toxicity at doses close to the normal therapeutic range.

### Gentamicin

Gentamicin is the most common agent requiring monitoring of serum levels. The ideal loading and maintenance dose is affected by age, weight, renal function and hydration. These can be calculated from a nomogram or computer program, assuming that the patient is in a steady state. The normal dosing interval is 8 h. Levels should always be checked around 24–48 h after commencing treatment, and intermittently thereafter:

- predose level: immediately before dose
- postdose level: 1 h after dose (either i.v. or i.m.).

If the first measured levels are out of range predose: 0.5–2 µg/ml, postdose: 5–8 µg/ml), carry out the following measures:

- Check there are no preanalytical reasons for result.
- Check the patient still needs an antibiotic.
- Check the patient still needs an aminoglycoside.
- Advise adjusting either total dose or dose interval.

Both high pre and postdose levels carry a risk of toxic effects. A high predose indicates drug accumulation, whereas a high postdose reflects an excessive total drug load. Common preanalytical reasons for out-of-range results are summarised in Table 3.2.

Once-daily dosage regimens have been developed to improve the convenience and reduce toxicity of gentamicin use. In a recent meta-analysis there was no significant impact on toxicity. Also daily regimens should not be used in clinical settings where the time of administration and post-dose level cannot be guaranteed.

### Tobramycin

This is rarely used, but same levels and dosage apply as for gentamicin.

### Amikacin

Amikacin is occasionally used on the advice of a microbiologist to treat nosocomial infection caused by an antibiotic resistant strain. Note that:

---

**TABLE 3.2   Preanalytical reasons for out-of-range results**

**Low**

Patient did not receive dose

Initial loading dose not given

Sample taken late

**High**

Sample taken from blocked infusion line

Sample collected with syringe used to give dose

Postdose sample collected too early

**Very high result**

If unexpected, often erroneous result

Check by rerunning specimen with positive and negative controls

If controls are correct, request further specimen of venous blood *by venipuncture*

---

- dose interval when renal function is normal: 12–18 h.
- predose level: 5–10 µg/ml
- postdose level: 20–25 µg/ml, taken 1 h after dose (as gentamicin).

## Vancomycin

This is the most commonly used glycopeptide antibiotic, and is used with increasing frequency for infections caused by resistant strains of *Staphylococcus aureus* and streptococci. Note that:

- dose interval when renal function is normal: 12 h
- predose level: 5–10 µg/ml
- postdose level: 20–40 µg/ml, at end of 1 h infusion.

In general it is advisable to avoid the peak level going over 50 µg/ml. The predose level is less significant as an indicator of potential toxicity, but is still useful, e.g. before giving a further dose in a patient with acute renal failure.

## Flucytosine

An antifungal agent used in combination with amphotericin B for serious, systemic yeast infections. There is a risk of bone marrow suppression, vomiting, diarrhoea and hepatotoxicity with high serum levels and prolonged courses. Note that:

- dose interval when renal function normal: 6 h
- predose level: 25–50 µg/ml
- postdose level: 80–100 µg/ml, 2 h after end of dose.

Nephrotoxicity is not a problem with flucytosine, but renal failure increases the risk of toxic effects.

# CONTROL, CONTAINMENT AND NOTIFICATION

# INFECTION CONTROL GUIDELINES

## PRESUMPTIVE MEASURES FOR SUSPECTED INFECTIONS

These are summarised in Table 4.1. A detailed explanation of the terms
standard, contact, airborne and droplet precautions can be found below.

 Control measures recommended in Table 4.1 below should always be
used in combination with standard precautions, e.g. a patient with
diarrhoea will require contact and standard precautions.

**TABLE 4.1   Presumptive measures for suspected infections**

| Problem | Precautions |
| --- | --- |
| Diarrhoea; incontinent of faeces or recent antibiotics | Contact |
| Meningitis | Droplet |
| Rash | |
| maculopapular, coryza and fever | Airborne |
| petechiae/ecchmoses and fever | Droplet |
| vesicular | Airborne and contact |
| Respiratory infection | |
| cough, fever and upper lobe shadow, HIV positive | Airborne |
| cough, fever and any lung infiltrate, HIV risk | Airborne |
| paroxysmal or severe/persistent cough during pertussis season | Droplet |
| infants and young children, especially bronchiolitis and croup | Contact |
| Risk of multidrug resistant organisms | |
| history of infection or colonisation | Contact |
| skin, wound, UTI after recent stay in unit with known resistance problem | Contact |
| Skin or wound infection | |
| abscess, draining wound that cannot be covered | Contact |

## MEASURES FOR CONFIRMED INFECTIONS

**TABLE 4.2   Measures for confirmed infections**

| Infection/condition | Precautions |
| --- | --- |
| Abscess | |
|    dressings cannot cover/contain exudate | Contact and standard |
|    dressings cover/contain exudate | Standard |
| AIDS | Standard |
| Actinomycosis | Standard |
| Adenovirus infection in infants/young children | Droplet, contact and standard |
| Amoebiasis | Standard |
| Anthrax | Standard |
| Antibiotic-associated colitis | Contact and standard |
| Antibiotic resistance, multiple | |
|    gastrointestinal | Contact and standard, until culture negative |
|    respiratory | Contact and Standard, until culture negative |
|    (pneumococcal) | Standard |
|    skin, wound, burn | Contact and standard, until culture negative |
| Arbovirus encephalitis | Standard |
| Arbovirus fevers | Standard |
| Ascaris infection | Standard |
| Aspergillosis | Standard |
| Babesiosis | Standard |
| Blastomycosis | Standard |
| Botulism | Standard |
| Brochiolitis in infants or young children | Contact and standard, duration of illness |
| Brucellosis | Standard |
| Campylobacter gastroenteritis | |
|    incontinent patients | Contact and standard |
|    infants in nappies | Contact and standard |
|    continent adults | Standard |
| Candidiasis, all forms | Standard |
| Catscratch fever | Standard |
| Cellulitis, uncontrolled drainage | Contact and standard, duration of illness |
| Chancroid | Standard |
| Chickenpox | Airbone, contact and standard |
| *Chlamydia trachomatis* | Standard |
| Cholera | |
|    incontinent patients | Contact and standard |
|    infants in nappies | Contact and standard |
|    continent adults | Standard |

**TABLE 4.2   Measures for confirmed infections (cont'd)**

| | |
|---|---|
| *Closed space infection, whether drained or not* | Standard |
| *Clostridium botulinum* | Standard |
| *Clostridium difficile* | Contact and standard |
| *Clostridium perfringens* | |
|    food poisoning | Standard |
|    gas gangrene | Standard |
| Congenital rubella | Contact and standard |
| Conjunctivitis | |
|   bacterial | |
|      Chlamydia | Standard |
|      gonococcal | Standard |
|      other | Standard |
|   viral | Contact and standard, duration of illness |
| Coxsackievirus | |
|   incontinent patients | Contact and standard |
|   infants in nappies | Contact and standard |
|   continent adults | Standard |
| Creuzfeldt-Jakob Disease | Seek advice from infection control team |
| Croup | Contact and contact, duration of illness |
| Cryptococcosis | Standard |
| Cryptosporidium | |
|   incontinent patients | Contact and standard |
|   infants in nappies | Contact and standard |
|   continent adults | Standard |
| Cysticercosis | Standard |
| Cytomegalovirus | Standard |
| Decubitus ulcer | |
|   dressings cannot cover/contain exudate | Contact and standard |
|   dressings cover/contain exudate | Standard |
| Dengue | Standard |
| Diarrhoea, acute | |
|   incontinent patients | Contact and standard |
|   infants in nappies | Contact and standard |
|   continent adults | Standard |
| Diphtheria | |
|   cutaneous | Contact and standard, until culture negative |
|   pharyngeal | Droplet and Standard, until culture negative |
| Ebola viral haemorrhagic fever | Seek immediate advice from infection control team |
| Echinococcus | Standard |
| Echovirus | |
|   incontinent patients | Contact and standard |
|   infants in nappies | Contact and standard |
|   continent adults | Standard |
| Encephalitis | See specific agents |
| Endometritis | Standard |
| Enterobiasis (pinworm) | Standard |

**TABLE 4.2  Measures for confirmed infections (cont'd)**

| | |
|---|---|
| *Enteroviral infections* | |
| incontinent patients | Contact and standard, duration of illness |
| infants in nappies | Contact and standard, duration of illness |
| continent adults | Standard |
| Epiglottitis, due to *H. influenzae* | Droplet and standard |
| Epstein–Barr virus | Standard |
| Erythema infectiosum (parvovirus B19) | Standard |
| *E. coli* enterocolitis | |
| incontinent patients | Contact and standard |
| infants in nappies | Contact and standard |
| continent adults | Standard |
| Food poisoning, all forms due to toxins | Standard |
| Furuncle (boil), infants and young children | Contact and standard, duration of illness |
| Gas Gangrene | Standard |
| Gastroenteritis; campylobacter, cholera, *E. coli*, giardia, rotavirus, salmonella (including *S. typhi*), shigella, others | |
| incontinent patients | Contact and standard |
| infants in nappies | Contact and standard |
| continent adults | standard |
| *Clostridium difficile* | Contact and standard |
| German measles | Droplet and standard |
| Giardia | |
| incontinent patients | Contact and standard |
| infants in nappies | Contact and standard |
| continent adults | Standard |
| Gonococcal ophthalmia neonatorum | Standard |
| Gonorrhoea | Standard |
| Group A streptococcal infection | |
| skin, wound or burn dressing cannot cover/contain exudate | Contact and standard, to 24hr after starting treatment |
| dressings cover/contain exudate | Standard |
| endometritis (puerperal sepsis) | Standard |
| pharyngitis, infants and young children | Droplet and standard, to 24hr after starting treatment |
| pneumonia, infants and young children | Droplet and standard, to 24hr after starting treatment |
| scarlet fever, infants and young children | Standard |
| Group B streptococcal infection, neonates | Standard |
| Granuloma inguinale | Standard |
| Guillain–Barre syndrome | Standard |
| Hand, foot and mouth disease | |
| incontinent patients | Contact and standard |
| infants in nappies | Contact and standard |
| continent adults | Standard |
| Hantavirus lung syndrome | Standard |
| *Helicobacter pylori* | Standard |

**TABLE 4.2   Measures for confirmed infections (cont'd)**

| | |
|---|---|
| Haemorrhagic fevers (Congo-Crimean, Ebola, Lassa, Marburg) | Seek immediate advice from infection control team |
| **Hepatitis, viral** | |
| hepatitis A | |
| incontinent patients | Contact and standard |
| infants in nappies | Contact and standard |
| continent adults | Standard |
| hepatitis B, HBsAg positive | Standard |
| hepatitis C and other non-A, non-B | Standard |
| **Herpangina** | |
| incontinent patients | Contact and standard |
| infants in nappies | Contact and standard |
| continent adults | Standard |
| **Herpes simplex** | |
| encephalitis | Standard |
| neonatal if mother has active infection and membranes ruptured for more than 4–6 hours, irrespective of route of delivery | Contact and standard |
| mucocutaneous, disseminated or severe | Contact and standard |
| mucocutaneous, recurrent skin, oral or genital | Standard |
| **Herpes zoster (varicella-zoster)** | |
| localised in immunocompromised patient, or disseminated | Airborne, contact and standard |
| localised in normal patient | Standard |
| Histoplasmosis | Standard |
| HIV | Standard |
| Hookworm | Standard |
| Human immunodeficiency virus | Standard |
| Impetigo | Contact and standard, to 24hr after starting antibiotics |
| Infectious mononucleosis | Standard |
| Influenza | Droplet and standard |
| Lassa fever | Seek immediate advice from infection control team |
| Legionnaires' disease | Standard |
| Leprosy | Standard |
| Leptospirosis | Standard |
| Lice | Contact and standard, to 24hr after starting treatment |
| Lyme disease | Standard |
| Lymphocytic choriomeningitis | Standard |
| Lymphogranuloma venereum | Standard |
| Malaria | Standard |
| Marburg virus infection | Seek immediate advice of infection control team |

**TABLE 4.2    Measures for confirmed infections (*cont'd*)**

| | |
|---|---|
| Measles, all forms | Airborne and standard |
| Melioidosis, all forms | Standard |
| Meningitis | |
| fungal | Standard |
| Gram negative bacillary in neonates | Standard |
| Haemophilus | Droplet and standard, to 24hr after starting antibiotics |
| meningococcal | Droplet and standard, to 24hr after starting therapy |
| Listeria | Standard |
| pneumococcal | Standard |
| tuberculous | Standard, if no evidence of lung disease |
| Meningococcal septicaemia | Droplet and standard, to 24hr after starting antibiotics |
| Molluscum contagiosum | Standard |
| Mucormycosis | Standard |
| Multiple antibiotic resistance | |
| gastrointestinal | Contact and standard, until culture negative |
| respiratory | Contact and standard, until culture negative |
| (pneumococcal) | Standard |
| skin, wound, burn | Contact and standard, until culture negative |
| Mumps | Droplet and standard |
| Mycobacteria, nontuberculous, pulmonary and wound | Standard |
| *Mycoplasma pneumonia* | Droplet and standard, duration of illness |
| Necrotising enterocolitis | Standard |
| Nocardiosis | Standard |
| Norwalk agent gastroenteritis | |
| incontinent patients | Contact and standard |
| infants in nappies | Contact and standard |
| continent adults | Standard |
| Orf | Standard |
| Parainfluenza virus (infants and young children) | Contact and standard, duration of illness |
| Parvovirus B19 | Droplet and standard, see infection control for details |
| Pediculosis | Contact and standard, to 24hr after starting treatment |
| Pertussis | Droplet and standard, to 5d after starting treatment |
| Pinworm | Standard |
| Plague | |
| bubonic | Standard |
| pneumonic | Droplet and standard, to 72hr after starting treatment |
| Pneumonia | |
| adenovirus | Droplet, contact and standard |
| *Burkholderia cepacia* in cystic fibrosis | Seek infection control advice |
| Chlamydia | Standard |

**TABLE 4.2  Measures for confirmed infections (cont'd)**

| | |
|---|---|
| fungal | Standard |
| *Haemophilus influenzae* | |
| adults | Standard |
| children, any age | Droplet and standard, to 24hr after starting treatment |
| Legionella | Standard |
| meningococcal | Droplet and standard, to 24hr after starting treatment |
| Mycoplasma | Droplet and standard, for duration of illness |
| *Pneumocystis carinii* | Standard, avoid placing with immunocompromised patient |
| *Staphylococcus aureus* | Standard |
| streptococcus group A | |
| adult | Standard |
| children | Droplet and standard, to 24hr after starting treatment |
| viral:adult | Standard |
| viral:children | Contact and standard, for duration of illness |
| Polio | Standard |
| Psittacosis | Standard |
| Q fever | Standard |
| Rabies | Standard |
| Ratbite fever | Standard |
| Relapsing fever | Standard |
| Resistance, multiple antibiotic | |
| gastrointestinal | Contact and standard, until culture negative |
| respiratory | Contact and standard, until culture negative |
| (pneumococcal) | Standard |
| skin, wound, burn | Contact and standard, until culture negative |
| Respiratory infection, acute (not covered elsewhere) | |
| adults | Standard |
| young children | Contact and standard, for duration of illness |
| Respiratory syncytial virus | |
| infants and young children | Contact and standard, for duration of illness |
| immunocompromised adults | Contact and standard, for duration of illness |
| Reye's syndrome | Standard |
| Rheumatic fever | Standard |
| Rickettsial fevers | Standard |
| Ringworm | Standard |
| Ritter's disease | |
| (staphylococcal scalded skin syndrome) | Standard |
| Roseola infantum (exanthem subitum) | Standard |
| Rotavirus infection | |
| incontinent patients | Contact and standard |
| infants in nappies | Contact and standard |
| continent adults | Standard |

## TABLE 4.2 Measures for confirmed infections (cont'd)

| | |
|---|---|
| Rubella | Droplet and standard, until 7 days after onset of rash |
| Salmonella (including *S. typhi*) | |
|   incontinent patients | Contact and standard |
|   infants in nappies | Contact and standard |
|   continent adults | Standard |
| Scabies | Contact and standard, to 24hr after starting treatment |
| Scalded skin syndrome, staphylococcal | Standard |
| Schistosomiasis (bilharzia) | Standard |
| Shigellosis | |
|   incontinent patients | Contact and standard |
|   infants in nappies | Contact and standard |
|   continent adults | Standard |
| Sporotrichosis | Standard |
| Staphylococcal infection | |
|   skin, wound or burn | |
|     dressing cannot cover/contain exudate | Contact and standard, for duration of infection |
|     dressings cover/contain exudate | Standard |
|   enterocolitis | |
|     incontinent patients | Contact and standard |
|     infants in nappies | Contact and standard |
|     continent adults | Standard |
|   methicillin resistant | See local policy |
|   pneumonia | Standard |
|   scalded skin syndrome | Standard |
|   toxic shock syndrome | Standard |
| Streptococcal infection (group A strep.) | |
|   skin, wound or burn | |
|     dressing cannot cover/contain exudate | Contact and standard, to 24hr after starting treatment |
|     dressings cover/contain exudate | Standard |
|   endometritis (puerperal sepsis) | Standard |
|   pharyngitis, infants and young children | Droplet and standard, to 24hr after starting treatment |
|   pneumonia, infants and young children | Droplet and standard, to 24hr after starting treatment |
|   scarlet fever, infants and young children | Standard |
| Streptococcal infection (group B), neonates | Standard |
| Streptococcal infection (other groups) | Standard |
| Strongyloidiasis | Standard |
| Syphilis, all forms | Standard |
| Tapeworm, all types | Standard |
| Tetanus | Standard |
| Tinea | Standard |

**TABLE 4.2 Measures for confirmed infections (*cont'd*)**

| | |
|---|---|
| Toxoplasmosis | Standard |
| Toxic shock syndrome | Standard |
| Trachoma, acute | Standard |
| Trench mouth (Vincent's angina) | Standard |
| Trichinosis | Standard |
| Trichomoniasis | Standard |
| Trichuris (whipworm) | Standard |
| Tuberculosis | |
| extrapulmonary | Standard |
| laryngeal | Airborne and standard |
| | Until smear negative and improving on therapy |
| pulmonary | Airborne and standard |
| | Until smear negative and improving on therapy |
| Typhoid fever | |
| incontinent patients | Contact and standard |
| infants in nappies | Contact and standard |
| continent adults | Standard |
| Typhus | Standard |
| Urinary tract infection | Standard |
| Varicella (chickenpox) | Airborne, contact and standard |
| Vincent's angina (trench mouth) | Standard |
| Whooping cough (pertussis) treatment | Droplet and standard, to 5d after starting |
| Wound infections | |
| dressing cannot cover/contain exudate | Contact and standard, for duration of infection |
| dressings cover/contain exudate | Standard |
| *Yersinia enterocolitica* gastroenteritis | |
| disseminated | Airborne, contact and standard, duration of infection |
| immunocompromised patient, localised | Airborne, contact and standard, duration of infection |
| immunocompetent patient, localised | Standard |
| Zygomycosis | Standard |
| Zoster (varicella-zoster) | Airborne, contact and standard |

## STANDARD PRECAUTIONS

### When?

At all times, by all staff, and for all patients. Standard precautions apply to blood, all body fluids (except sweat), mucous membranes and damaged skin.

### What?

- Wash hands after contact with above body fluids or surfaces, immediately after removing gloves, and if necessary between procedures involving the same patient. Decontamination with an alcohol hand rub is an acceptable alternative, if hands are aesthetically clean after contact with a dry body surface.
- Put on clean gloves before contact with mucous membranes, damaged skin surfaces, blood, body fluids, secretions, excretions, or contaminated objects. Change gloves between procedures on the same patient if in contact with substances likely to contain many microorganisms. Remove gloves immediately after use and wash hands before touching noncontaminated surfaces or objects.
- Wear a mask and eye protection (goggles or face shield) during procedures that may splash or spray blood, body fluids or secretions.
- Also wear a disposable plastic apron or disposable gown to protect clothing and body surfaces against splashes of blood or body fluids. Wash hands carefully after removal of apron or tabard.
- Used patient-care equipment soiled with blood, body fluids or secretions should also be handled as if contaminated. Reusable devices must not be reused until they have been properly cleaned and prepared for reuse.
- The patient's immediate environment and any adjacent surfaces likely to be touched by attending healthcare staff should be regularly cleaned and disinfected.
- Contamination of clothing or transfer to other patients or their immediate environment should be avoided during handling or transport of soiled linen.
- Every effort should be made to avoid sharp or needlestick injuries. Do not attempt to recap needles using both hands, or by pointing the needle tip towards any part of the body. Do not remove needles from syringes by hand. All sharp instruments should be discarded into a puncture-resistant container. Whenever the need for resuscitation can be predicted, use a mouthpiece or resuscitation bag instead of a mouth-to-mouth technique.
- Patients likely to deliberately contaminate the immediate environment or who show substantial evidence of a lack of personal hygiene should be placed in a single-bed sideward, if available.

## CONTACT PRECAUTIONS

### When?

Contact precautions are used, in addition to standard precautions, for any infections transmitted by direct or indirect contact with the patients and their immediate environment.

### What?

- The patient should be in a single-bed sideward, if available. If not, patients should be grouped (cohorted) in a room with other patients who have the same infection, and no other.
- In addition to standard precautions put on gloves before entering the patient's room and if your clothing may touch the patient or the immediate surroundings, put on a plastic apron or disposable gown as well. These should be removed immediately before leaving the patient's environment.
- Movement and transport of the patient outside the room should be restricted to essential purposes only.
- Restrict the use of non-critical care equipment to a single patient, if possible. If not, then adequately clean and disinfect before use for a further patient.

## AIRBORNE PRECAUTIONS

### When?

Airborne precautions should be used, in addition to standard precautions, to prevent transmission of any infections spread via airborne droplet nuclei which can be dispersed widely by air currents in a room.

### What?

- Where available, the patient should be placed in a single-bed sideward with negative pressure ventilation. Ventilation should deliver 6–12 air changes per hour and either discharge outside, or if recirculated to the hospital it should be filtered first. If no sidewards are available, cohort patients with the same and no other infection.
- A conventional theatre mask should be worn as respiratory protection when entering the room, except in the case of measles-immune staff entering the room of a patient with measles, or varicella-immune staff entering a varicella-infected patient's room. Staff susceptible to either measles or varicella should not enter the room of patients known or suspected to have either infection, if it can be avoided.
- Restrict the movement of the patient outside the room to essential purposes. While outside the room, the patient should wear a surgical mask.

 There are additional measures specific to the prevention of tuberculosis. Further precautions will be required in healthcare settings where tuberculosis is common, or where multidrug resistant tuberculosis can be anticipated.

## DROPLET PRECAUTIONS

### When?
Droplet precautions are used, as well as standard precautions, to prevent any infections transmitted in the large droplets generated by the patient during coughing, sneezing, talking and some procedures.

### What?

- The patient should be in a single-bed sideward, or failing that cohorted with other patients who have the same but no other infection. If that is not possible, a 3ft gap should be kept between the patient and other patients and visitors. Special ventilation systems are not necessary.
- Wear a theatre mask when working within 3ft of the patient, and when the patient has to be moved out of the room, place a surgical mask on the patient to reduce dispersal of droplets.

---

**Practice note**
There are bound to be variations in local infection control practice, dictated by differences in health care resources and epidemiological priorities. If in doubt, check your local infection control policy and refer to the original HICPAC publication. Reprints can be obtained from Mailstop E-69, Hospital Infections Program, National Center for Infectious Diseases, Centers for Disease Control and Prevention, Atlanta, GA 30333, USA.

---

These guidelines are based on the Guideline for Isolation Precautions in Hospitals (Garner JS, Hospital Infection Control Practices Advisory Committee 1996 Infection Control and Hospital Epidemiology 17: 53–80) and were adapted for use in the Royal Shrewsbury Hospital by members of the infection control team there.

# INCUBATION PERIODS AND INFECTIVITY

These are summarised in Table 4.3.

**TABLE 4.3    Incubation periods and infectivity of common infections**

| Condition | Incubation period and infectivity |
| --- | --- |
| AIDS | Variable |
| antibody response | 1–3 months |
| HIV infection — AIDS | 2 months – > 10 years |
| infectivity | Unknown, ? from onset of infection, throughout life |
| Actinomycosis | Irregular |
| after oral colonisation | Probably years |
| after tissue trauma | Days or months |
| Amoebiasis | Often 2–4 weeks, range: a few days to years |
| infective | As long as cysts passed in faeces |
| Anisakiasis | |
| gastric symptoms | Within hours |
| bowel symptoms | days to weeks |
| Anthrax | Usually within 2 days, range: hours to 7 days |
| Arbovirus disease | 1–15 days, depending on type |
| arthritis & rash | 3–11 days |
| encephalitides | 5–15 days, mosquito-borne |
| | 7–14 days, tick-borne |
| fevers | 2–12 days, mosquito-borne |
| | 4–5 days, tick-borne |
| | 3–6 days, phlebotomine-borne |
| haemorrhagic fevers | 3–12 days |
| Ascariasis | 4–8 weeks to completion of life cycle |
| infective | As long as fertile female worms in intestine |
| Aspergillosis | Probably days to weeks |
| Babesiosis | 1 week to 12 months |
| infective | In asymptomatic blood donors for up to 12 months |
| Bartonellosis | 16–22 days, up to 3–4 months |
| bacteria may persist in blood for years after infection | |
| Blastomycosis | Median = 45 days, range: weeks to months |
| Botulism | |
| adult | 12–36 hours |
| wound | 4–14 days |
| Brucellosis | Highly variable, usually 5–60 days |
| Campylobacter | 2–5 days, range: 1–10 days |
| infective | For duration of infection, 2–7 wk if not treated |
| Candida, oral | 2–5 days, variable |
| infective | Probably as long as lesions persist |

**TABLE 4.3    Incubation periods and infectivity of common infections (cont'd)**

| | |
|---|---|
| Catscratch disease | Variable |
|   papule | 3–14 days |
|   lymph nodes | 5 days to 7 weeks |
| Chancroid | 3–14 days |
|   infectivity | Until healed, or 1–2 wk after starting treatment |
| Chickenpox | 10–21 days, usually 14–17 days |
|   perinatal | Shorter period, usually 14–17 days |
|   infectivity | 1–2 days before rash to 5 days after last new crop of vesicles or all vesicles crusted over |
| Chlamydias | |
|   *C. pneumoniae* | > 10 days |
|   *C. psittaci* | 5–21 days |
|   *C. trachomatis* | |
|     genital | Around 7–14 days |
|     conjunctivitis | 5–14 days |
|     pneumonia | 4–6 weeks |
| Cholera | Usually 2–3 days, range: hours to 5 days |
| Clostridial myonecrosis | 1–4 days, range: 6 hours to 3 weeks |
| Clostridial (*C. perfringens*) food poisoning | 7–15 hours, Range 6–24 hours |
| *Clostridium botulinum* | 12–36 hours, range 8 hours to 8 days |
| Common cold | Usually 2 days, range 12 hours to 5 days |
|   infective | From 24hr before to 5d after onset |
| Conjunctivitis | |
|   adenovirus | 4–12 days |
|     infectivity | Late incubation period–14 days after onset |
|   *C. trachomatis* | 5–12 days, range: 3d–6wk newborn, 6–19d adult |
|     infective | While genital or eye infection persists |
|   *N. gonorrhoeae* | 1–5 days |
|   other bacteria | 1–3 days |
| Cryptosporidiosis | Average 7 days, range around 1–12 days |
|   infective | From onset until 2 weeks after symptoms resolve |
| Cytomegalovirus | |
|   (blood borne) | 3–8 weeks after transfusion |
|   during birth | 3–12 weeks after delivery |
|     infectivity | Virus in urine and saliva for months after infection. Shorter persistance in adults, latency more common |
| Dengue fever | 5–7 days, range: 3–14 days |
| Dermatophytoses | |
|   tinea barbae, capitis | Around 10–14 days |
|   tinea corporis, cruris | 4–10 days |
|   infective | As long as lesions persist |
| Diphtheria | Usually 2–5 days |
|   infective | For 2–4 wk, or shortly after starting therapy |

**TABLE 4.3   Incubation periods and infectivity of common infections (cont'd)**

| | |
|---|---|
| Diphyllobothrium | 3–6 weeks |
| Dracunculiasis | Around 12 months |
| Ebola haemorrhagic fever | 2–21 days |
| infective | As long as blood and secretions contain virus |
| Ehrlichiosis | 1–3 weeks |
| Enterobiasis | 2–6 weeks to complete worm life cycle |
| infective | As long as worms discharge eggs on perianal skin |
| Enteric virus infection | Usually 3–5 days, range 2 days to 6 weeks |
| adenovirus | 8–10 days |
| astrovirus | 1–2 days |
| calicivirus | 1–3 days |
| Norwalk virus | 12–48 hours |
| infective | Up to 48hr after diarrhoea stops |
| rotavirus | 1–3 days |
| infective | Until 8th day of infection, longer if immunocompromised |
| Gastroenteritis | |
| E. coli | 10–72 hours |
| infective | While bacteria excreted, up to several weeks |
| salmonella | 6 hours to 3 days |
| infective | throughout infection, sometimes carrier state |
| shigella | 1–3 days |
| infective | While bacteria in faeces, usually around 4 wk |
| viral | 3–5 days |
| infectivity | Depends on specific aetiology |
| Erysipeloid | 2–7 days |
| Erythema infectiosum | 4–20 days |
| infective | Until rash appears |
| Escherichia coli enteritis | |
| infective | While present in faeces |
| EHEC | 12–60 hours |
| infective | Up to 3wk in 33% children |
| EIEC | 10–18 hours, or more |
| EPEC | Adults, 9–12 hours or more |
| ETEC | Adults, 10–72 hours |
| Food poisoning | |
| B. cereus | |
| emetic | 1–6 hours |
| diarrhoeal | 6–24 hours |
| C. perfringens | 10–12 hours, range 6–24 hours |
| S. aureus | Usually 2–4 hours; range 1/2–7hr |
| Giardiasis | 5–> 25 days |
| infective | Throughout infection, up to several months |
| Glandular fever | 4–6 weeks |
| infectivity | Up to over 1 year after infection |
| Gonococcal ophthalmitis | 1–5 days |
| infective | For 24hr after starting treatment |

**TABLE 4.3    Incubation periods and infectivity of common infections (cont'd)**

| | |
|---|---|
| Gonococcal infection | Usually 2–7 days, sometimes longer |
|    infectivity | Ends hours after starting treatment |
| Granuloma inguinale | 1 week to 3 months |
|    infective | Probabaly for duration of open lesions |
| Haemolytic uraemic syndrome | Usually 3–4, up to 10 days |
|    infective | Up to 3 wk in 33% children, after EHEC diarrhoea |
| Hand, foot & mouth | 3–5 days |
|    virus persists in faeces for several weeks | |
| Hepatitis A | Average 28–30 days, range 15–45 days |
|    infectivity | Last half of period to 7 days after onset of jaundice |
| Hepatitis B | Average 60–90 days, range 45–180 days |
|    infectivity | Greater if surface and e antigens present |
| Hepatitis C | Usually 6–9 weeks, range 2 weeks to 6 months |
| Herpes simplex | |
|    anogenital | 2–12 days |
|       infective | 7–12d after primary lesion |
| | Repeated reactivation, sometimes asymptomatic |
|    neonatal | 2–28 days |
|    childhood | 2–14 days |
| Histoplasmosis | 3–14 days |
| Infectious mononucleosis | 4–6 weeks |
|    infectivity | Up to over 1 year after infection |
| Influenza | 1–5 days |
|    infectivity | 3–5 days from clinical onset; children: 7 days |
| Invasive helminth | Usually within 3 months |
|    strongyloides | Up to many years later |
| Lassa fever | 6–21 days |
|    infectivity | Urine 3–9 weeks from onset, saliva during fever |
| Legionnaires' disease | |
|    adults | Usually 5–6 days, range 2–10 days |
|    Pontiac fever | Usually 24–48 hours, range 5–66 hours |
| Leishmaniasis | |
|    cutaneous | Several weeks to months |
|    visceral | 2–4 months, range 10 days to 2 years |
| Leprosy | Range 9 months to 20 years |
|    tuberculoid | Average 4 years |
|    lepromatous | Average 8 years |
|       infective | Up to 3 months after start of continuous treatment |
| Leptospirosis | 7–12 days, range 2–20 days |
| Listeriosis | 3–70 days in food-related outbreaks |

**TABLE 4.3    Incubation periods and infectivity of common infections (cont'd)**

| | |
|---|---|
| infective | Vaginal discharge in mothers of infected infants<br>For 7–10d after delivery, shed in faeces for months |
| Lyme disease | 3–32 days to erythema migrans |
| Lymphocytic choriomeningitis virus | 15–21 days |
| Malaria<br>*Plasmodium falciparum*<br>*Plasmodium vivax & ovale*<br>*Plasmodium malariae* | Depends on spp.<br>12 days approx.<br>14 days approx.<br>30 days approx. |

| Onset | Falciparum | others |
|---|---|---|
| < 1 month | 90% | 25% |
| 1–4 months | 10% | 30% |
| > 6 months | < 1% | 35% |
| > 12 months | | 10% |

| | |
|---|---|
| Measles<br><br>infective | 7–14 days, adults usually > children<br>About 10 days to fever, 14 days to rash onset<br>Just before prodrome to 4d after rash onset |
| Melioidosis | 2 days to several years after injury<br>May remain latent up to 26 years |
| Meningococcal meningitis<br>infective | Usually 3–4 days, range 2–10 days<br>For around 24hr after starting treatment |
| Molluscum contagiosum<br>infective | 7 days to 6 months<br>Probably as long as lesions persist |
| Mumps<br>infective | 12–25 days<br>From 12th–25th day after exposure |
| Mycobacteria, atypical | Weeks to months |
| *Mycoplasma pneumoniae*<br>infective | 6–23 days<br>Up to 20d or longer, persists despite treatment |
| Parvovirus<br>infective | 4–20 days<br>Until rash appears |
| Pertussis<br>infective<br><br>infectivity | 7–14 days<br>From early catarrhal stage to 3wk after paroxysms<br>Ceases after approx. 5d erythromycin treatment |
| Pinta<br>potentially infective | 7–21 days<br>While active lesions |
| Plague<br>bubonic<br>pneumonic<br>    may be communicated directly | <br>2–6 days<br>1–6 days |
| Pneumococcal pneumonia<br>infective | Unclear; around 1–3 days<br>Up to 24–48hr after starting penicillin |

**TABLE 4.3    Incubation periods and infectivity of common infections (cont'd)**

| | |
|---|---|
| Polio | |
|    wild virus | 9–12 days, range 5–35 days |
|    vaccine recipient | 7–28 days |
|    vaccine contact | 7–60 days |
|    infective | A few days before clinical infection, virus in faeces for up to 3 wk after symptoms |
| Poxvirus | Variable, 2 weeks to 6 months |
| Prion disease | |
|    brain inoculation | 18–54 months |
|    muscle inoculation | 5–20 years |
|    ingestion | > 4 years |
| Psittacosis | 4–15 days |
| Q fever | 14–39 days |
| Rabies | 20–60 days, range 4 days to 19 years. Depends on dose, proximity to brain. Virus travels at 12–24 mm/day via axons |
| Ratbite fever | 3–10 days |
| Relapsing fever | 5–15 days |
| Respiratory syncytial virus | 2–8 days |
|    infective | Just before and during infection, rarely for weeks |
| Rhinovirus infection | Usually 2 days, range 12 hours to 5 days |
|    infective | From 24hr before to 5d after onset |
| Rocky mountain spotted fever | 2–14 days |
| Rotavirus | 1–3 days |
|    infective | Until 8th day of infection, longer if immunocompromised |
| Rubella | Usually 16–18 days, range 12–23 days |
|    infective | For 1 wk before to 4d after rash, continued virus excretion for months in congenital syndrome |
| Salmonella | 6 hours to 3 days, depending on dose |
|    infective | Throughout infection, sometimes carrier state |
| Scabies | 2–6 weeks, first time; 1–4 days afterwards |
|    infective | Until mites and eggs destroyed after 1–2 treatments |
| Schistosomiasis | 2–6 weeks after exposure (Katayama fever) |
| Shigellosis | 1–3 days |
|    infective | While bacteria in faeces, usually around 4wk |
| Staphylococcal infection | |
|    food poisoning | 2–6 hours |
|    impetigo | 1–10 days |
|    scalded skin syndrome | 1–10 days |
|    infective | While lesions discharge or while carrier state |
| Streptococcal infection | |
|    pharyngitis | 2–4 days |

**TABLE 4.3    Incubation periods and infectivity of common infections (cont'd)**

| | |
|---|---|
| impetigo | 7–10 days |
| infective | 10–21 days untreated, treated: 24hr |
| Syphilis | Around 3 weeks, range 3–90 days |
| Tetanus | 3 days to 3 weeks |
| | Depends on dose, and severity of injury |
| Threadworm | 2–6 weeks |
| Toxocariasis | |
| acute | Weeks to months |
| ocular granuloma | Up to 10 years |
| Toxoplasmosis | 10–23 days |
| Trichomoniasis | 4–20 days |
| infective | For duration of infection, may be years |
| Trypanosomiasis (African) | Around 5–14 days |
| Tuberculosis | 1–3 months (primary complex) |
| infective | As long as viable bacilli present in sputum |
| Tularaemia | 3–5 days, range 1–21 days |
| Typhoid fever | 5–21 days, depends on dose |
| infective | For at least 1 wk after convalescence |
| | 10% patients remain faeces positive for 3 months |
| | 2–5% patients become chronic carriers |
| Typhus | |
| epidemic | 1–2 weeks after bite |
| murine | 1–2 weeks |
| scrub | 10–12 days |
| Urethritis | |
| gonococcal, male | Usually 2–5 days, range 1–10 days |
| gonococcal, female | Most < 10 days |
| nonspecific | 7–14 days |
| *Vibrio parahaemolyticus* | 23 hours, range 5–92 hours |
| Viral haemorrhagic fever | 1 day to 6 weeks |
| yellow fever | 3–6 days |
| dengue | 2–7 days |
| Omsk haemorrhagic fever | 3–7 days |
| chickungunya | 1–12 days |
| Lassa fever | 3–16 days |
| junin | 2–6 days |
| machupo | 2–6 days |
| sabia | 2–6 days |
| Rift Valley fever | 3–12 days |
| Congo-Crimean haemorrhagic fever | 3–12 days |
| Hantaan virus | 2 weeks, range 5–42 days |
| Seoul virus | 2 weeks, range 5–42 days |
| Puumola virus | 2 weeks, range 5–42 days |
| Ebola fever | 5–10 days, range 2–19 days |
| Marburg fever | 5–10 days, range 2–19 days |

**TABLE 4.3    Incubation periods and infectivity of common infections (cont'd)**

| | |
|---|---|
| Warts | 2–3 months, range up to 2 years |
| Yaws | 2 weeks to 3 months |
|   infective | Variable while moist lesions present |
| Yellow fever | 3–6 days after bite |
| Yersiniosis | 1–14 days, usually 4–6 days |
| | Bacteria in faeces as long as symptoms persist |

Sources:

Beneson A (ed) 1995 *Control of communicable disease manual*, 16th edition. American Public Health Association, Washington, DC

Davies EG, Elliman DAC, Hart CA, Nicoll A, and Rudd P 1994 *Manual of Childhood Infections* WB Saunders & Co Ltd, London

Mandell GL et al 1995 *Mandell, Douglas and Bennett's Principles and Practice of Infectious Diseases* Churchill Livingstone, Edinburgh

# HAND HYGIENE

> Hand hygiene is both the single most important and the most neglected infection control measure practised by hospital staff.

### Rationale

Many of the common nosocomial pathogens (e.g. *S. aureus* and *Klebsiella* spp.) rely on the hands of hospital staff for transmission between patients. When faced with a time–space infection cluster, common-source incident or confirmed outbreak, control measures often start with improvements in staff hand hygiene. The increasing prevalence of multiple antibiotic resistant strains has resulted in renewed enthusiasm for infection control interventions, especially hand hygiene measures.

### Behaviour modification

Motivating hospital staff to wash their hands and comply with other hand hygiene measures is an uphill struggle, reflecting the difficulty of persuading individuals to maintain a high level of vigilance against something they cannot see, and will not encounter if their personal practice is consistently good. The more senior and experienced the staff, the more difficult it will be to change their practice. Yet it is the most experienced staff that provide the day-to-day role models for juniors to follow. Different grades and categories of staff will require different approaches if there is to be any beneficial effect. Your approach will also have to change with time, as staff become accustomed to your methods.

### How

The method taught should be consistent throughout the hospital, and easily practised by all grades of staff as second nature. A widely applied method was described by Ayliffe et al 1978 (J Clin Path 31: 923–8) involving eight steps. Key points are that:

- hands should be wet before applying disinfectant
- palms, interdigital spaces, thumbs, and dorsa should be rubbed repeatedly to lather
- cleansing agent should then be rinsed off
- and then the hands carefully dried.

Performed as described, the procedure should take no more than one minute (not suitable for surgical preoperative scrub-up).

## When

The handwash should take place before any contact with patients, in-between patient contact, and at the end of a working day or shift. It should be performed even when latex gloves are worn (a supplementary hygiene measure; not a substitute) and even if contact is with a dry body surface.

## What

Povidone iodine, chlorhexidine and alcoholic preparations are the most common choice. Preparations containing chlorhexidine are useful in situations where a prolonged effect is required. Alcohol gel handrub is a popular alternative in clinical settings where handwashing is difficult, but remember the poor effect of alcohols against enteric viruses.

## Problems

*Poor compliance* Are there enough washbasins in convenient locations? Are the elbow-operated taps easy to use? Is the water temperature too hot? Are staff developing skin reactions? Do staff dislike the disinfectant in use? Is there any disinfectant? Is there a choice of hand disinfectant? Are senior staff providing a satisfactory example?

*Skin reactions* Discover what technique staff are using. Are hands wet before applying disinfectant? Is too much disinfectant used? Is it being washed off properly? Are hands being dried thoroughly afterwards? Do they have access to a suitable emmolient? Have they tried another disinfectant wash or alcohol gel as an alternative?

*Bar soap* In theory this is suitable; in practice, it is often left in a puddle, therefore a potential node in the web of transmission; also it is inadequate against VRE. Are liquid soap dispensers available? Do staff bring in their own soap, or do they keep soap left by patients? Are hospital domestic staff instructed to restock washbasins with soap? Who brought in the soap dish!

*Senior staff* Investigate whether they are failing to set acceptable standards or to act as a satisfactory role model. Are they difficult to educate/resistant to change? How much real contact do they have with infection-control staff? If there is not much contact, whose fault is that? Do senior staff think infection control is only carried out by the infection-control team? How good is their compliance in other aspects of hospital hygiene?

# HOSPITAL WASTE DISPOSAL

With the loss of Crown immunity, hospitals in the UK have a legal responsibility to ensure safe disposal of waste. Hospital waste is colour coded to help separate waste that requires different methods of disposal. [Coding is according to DHSS HN (82) 22.]

## Categories of waste

- **A**: domestic (black bag). Is not in any other category.
- **B**: clinical (yellow bag). This is material contaminated with pathogens and designated for secure transit and incineration.
- **C**: sharps (sharps box; British Standard BS 7320, assessed by quality system BS EN ISO 9002 Quality Systems, UN 3291). This material requires secure disposal.
- **D**: human tissue (yellow bag). If identifiable, these go for immediate incineration, or storage in mortuary.
- **E**: laboratory waste. Cultures and specimens require autoclaving prior to disposal.

## Sewage

- Faeces, urine or waste water can be discharged to the domestic sewer, untreated, via a sluice.
- Avoid using sinks.
- Do not use disinfectant as this may destroy useful commensal bacteria.

# HYGIENE STANDARDS

## AIR QUALITY

In hospital practice, air is sampled to assess potential bacterial exposure in clean environments such as operating theatres. Two methods are commonly used: settle plates and the slit sampler. If settle plates are to be used, they should contain a nonselective medium such as blood agar. Sufficient plates should be left in positions of maximum air disturbance to produce interpretable results, and they should be exposed for at least 10–60 minutes. A slit sampler impels a known volume of air from the immediate aerial environment at a steady rate over the exposed surface of a rotating agar plate.

The precise infection risk of a measured number of airborne nosocomial pathogens is not known, but recommended air hygiene standards have been published as a basis for risk assessment ($\rightarrow$ Table 4.4)

**TABLE 4.4   Air quality standards**

| Setting | Standard |
| --- | --- |
| Filtered theatre input | $\leq 0.5$ bacteria/m$^3$ |
| Within 30 cm of operation site | $\leq 10$ bacteria/m$^3$ |
| Elsewhere | $\leq 20$ bacteria/m$^3$ |
| Plastic isolation bubble | $\leq 1$ bacterium/m$^3$ |

## WATER QUALITY

The quality of water can be assessed by its bacterial content. After chlorination 'Coliforms' should be undetectable in water entering a distribution system. A small amount of contamination is inevitable during passage through the system but this should still be minimal at the points where water is accessed. There should be no *E. coli* in any 100 ml sample ($\rightarrow$ Table 4.5). Coliforms should not be found in any two consecutive samples from the same outlet and in < 5% of 50 or more samples taken at intervals over one year.

When taking water samples, avoid contamination of the sterile container by environmental bacteria. Flame the taps and allow a free flow for 5 min. If immersing container, open it towards the flow at 30 cm depth with the hand downstream. Five litre samples are required for detection of *Legionella pneumophila*. Keep cool during delivery. Transit time should be less than 6 h.

**TABLE 4.5   Water quality standards**

| Standard | Coliforms/100 ml | E. coli/100 ml |
|---|---|---|
| Excellent | 0 | 0 |
| Satisfactory | 1–3 | 0 |
| Intermediate | 4–9 | 0 |
| Unsatisfactory | > 9 | > 0 |

As *E. coli* is the most common aerobe in the human intestine and has a relatively short environmental survival, its presence is a sensitive indicator of recent pollution with human or animal faeces. Enterococci are less common, but the association of different enterococcal species with domestic animals such as chickens and pigs may help trace a source of faecal pollution. *Clostridium perfringens* is sometimes used as an index or remote or intermittent pollution since it may survive in spore form when other bacterial indicators cannot.

# INSPECTIONS

## KITCHEN INSPECTION

Hospital kitchens are a potential source of food poisoning for the entire hospital. The increased susceptibility of patients to infection means that a very high standard of hygiene should be practised by hospital catering staff. It is the responsibility of the Infection Control Team to inspect hospital kitchens at least once a year, preferably in the company of a catering manager and senior maintenance engineer. A record should be kept of observations made, and a report provided for the Infection Control Committee.

A detailed checklist should cover the following aspects:

*Staff*

- Are they fit for work, trained for the job, familiar with hygiene regulations?
- Is there evidence of a high standard of personal hygiene?

*Raw materials/ingredients*

- Do these arrive in satisfactory condition?
- Are they stored separately from cooked food?
- Is low temperature storage accessible, large and cool enough?
- Is a stock record maintained?

*Procedures*

- Are preparation surfaces/equipment clean and intact?
- Do cooked items reach sufficient temperatures for long enough?
- What arrangements are there for dispensing portions?
- How are meals distributed to wards?
- What policy is taken on retaining food for testing?
- Is shelf life indicated for perishables, and implemented?

*Cleaning*

- How are work surfaces, cooking vessels and utensils cleaned?
- What is done with crockery and cutlery returned from wards?
- What is done with food and other waste?
- What measures are used to deal with kitchen pests?

 There are specific hygiene measures to reduce the microbiological hazards of using cook–chill catering systems, which should be consulted if cook–chill is used in your hospital.

## LAUNDRY INSPECTION

*Staff*

- Are they fit for work?
- Are they trained in use of equipment and knowledgable about hygiene precautions?
- Is there evidence of personal hygiene in practice?

*Reception*

- Is infected linen kept separate from other categories?
- Are handling facilities suitable for dealing with spills and is there a sharps procedure?

*Equipment*

- Is load temperature monitored on washers?
- Is adequacy of disinfection ever tested?

*Clean dispatch*

- Is clean linen kept separate from used linen?
- What measures are taken to keep it clean during transport?

### Laundry hygiene standards

Soiled hospital linen is a potential infection risk to patients and staff. There have been regulations to reduce this risk since the early 1970s. These were revised in 1987 in response to changes in fabrics used in hospital and in laundry practice [DHSS, 1987, HC(37)30: Hospital laundry arrangements for used and infected linen].

Laundry is classified as used, infected and heat-labile. Linen that has been in contact with patients with gastrointestinal infections, or open pulmonary tuberculosis, and bloodstained linen from HIV or HBV positive patients is infected. Linen infested with lice or fleas is treated as if it were infected.

Infected linen should be placed in a water-soluble or alginate bag, and this bag placed in an outer bag prior to transfer to the laundry. The load should be washed on a hot cycle, i.e. 65°C for at least 10 minutes, then heat dried and finished as normal.

### OPERATING THEATRE INSPECTION

 Shorter pre- and postoperative stays in hospital have focussed attention on the role of events in the perioperative period as a determinant of surgical wound infection.

Periodic inspection of operating theatres by infection control staff may help to avoid preventable infections.

*Who?* Infection control staff (preferably both medical and nursing, both male and female), and Theatre Manager at a minimum, and possibly a senior maintenance engineer.

*When?* Preferably during a normal working day.

*What?* A detailed checklist should cover the following aspects:

- Patients: reception, anterooms, theatres, recovery area.
- Staff: changing rooms, scrub area, theatres, rest area.
- Equipment: store, inuse areas, service/cleaning.
- Consumables: store, inuse areas, discard/disposal.
- Engineering: ventilation, airflow, humidity.
- Architecture: cleanable surfaces, structural integrity, access routes.

# NEEDLESTICK PROTOCOL

 Around 90% needlestick and sharp injuries in hospital go unreported: a missed opportunity for preventing potentially fatal occupational infections.

## Protocol

### First aid

1. Wash puncture site with soap and warm water.
2. Encourage bleeding, if possible.
3. Dry carefully.
4. Report to supervisor.

### Action at unit

5. Contact occupational health.
6. Review hepatitis B and HIV risk of patient.
7. Counsel patient regarding HIV test, if indicated.
8. Arrange venesection of patient.

### Action by occupational health department

9. Record detailed circumstances of sharp injury.
10. Check hepatitis B vaccination status of staff. If unvaccinated, commence Hepatitus B vaccine course and if patient is Hepatitis B positive, give 0.06 ml/kg HBIG i.m.
11. Offer counselling regarding HIV risk.
12. Arrange venesection of patient for baseline serum.
13. Arrange follow-up appointment at 6 months, or earlier if recipient is anxious.
14. Return details of incident to infection control team.

 **Risk of seroconversion following needlestick injury is:**
- circa 30% from Hepatitis B$_e$Ag positive patient
- circa 3% for hepatitis C positive patient
- circa 0.3% from HIV positive patient.

**If high risk of exposure, recipient should begin post exposure prophylaxis with antiretroviral agents commencing within 2 hours of injury.**

In areas of high HIV prevalence, hospitals may offer staff combination therapy (e.g. Zidovudine 200 mg t.d.s., Lamivudine 150 mg t.d.s. and Indinavin 800 t.d.s. for 4 weeks) following sharps injury. Check who is responsible for this service *before* you have to deal with high-risk exposure.

# NOTIFIABLE DISEASES

The doctor who diagnoses a notifiable infectious disease should contact the consultant in communicable disease control (CCDC). However, it is often the microbiologist who confirms the aetiological diagnosis. You should therefore liaise with the local CCDC, or alternative, on notifiable infections, particularly in cases of enteritis, dysentery, meningitis and tuberculosis. Asymptomatic carriers do not legally require notification, but informal liaison with the CCDC may help improve the efficiency of control measures.

Notification of infectious diseases to the proper medical authorities is not the same as informing the Communicable Diseases Surveillance Centre (CDSC) (Colindale, London). Information returned to CDSC forms part of the epidemiological monitoring of major infectious diseases in England and Wales and is reported monthly in the Communicable Disease Report (CDR). The CDSC list includes a number of conditions of national importance that are not on the notifiable list (→ Table 4.6).

| TABLE 4.6  Notifiable diseases | |
|---|---|
| *England & Wales* | *Local variations (annotate as indicated)* |
| Acute encephalitis | |
| Acute poliomyelitis | |
| Anthrax | |
| Cholera | |
| Diphtheria | |
| Dysentery | |
| Food poisoning (confirmed or suspected) | |
| Lassa fever | |
| Leprosy | |
| Leptospirosis | |
| Malaria | |
| Measles | |
| Meningitis | |
| Meningococcal septicaemia, without meningitis | |
| Mumps | |
| Ophthalmia neonatorum | |
| Paratyphoid fever | |
| Plague | |
| Rabies | |
| Relapsing fever | |
| Rubella | |

**TABLE 4.6   Notifiable diseases (cont'd)**

Scarlet fever

Smallpox

Tetanus

Tuberculosis; all forms

Typhoid fever

Typhus

Viral haemorrhagic fever (e.g. Ebola fever)

Viral hepatitis

Whooping cough

Yellow fever

## OUTBREAKS

### SUSPECTED OUTBREAK: INITIAL RESPONSE

If you are the first to respond to a suspected hospital outbreak, you have to steer a course between a premature reaction to a false alarm and missing the best opportunity to halt the spread of the outbreak before it gets out of hand.

There are three main aims:

1. confirmation of an outbreak
2. appropriate management of early cases.
3. alerting the infection control team.

- **Teamwork and effective communication is required from the start; do not try to manage it all by yourself.**
- **you are not trying to apportion blame.**

### Procedure

1. Establish a line of communication with reporting staff, giving name, status and contact number.
2. Ask for the following information:
   - How many patients?
   - Where are they?
   - What signs of infection have been noticed?
   - When did they develop signs of infection?
   - How long have they been in hospital?
3. Request collection of relevant diagnostic specimens.
4. Ask for the name and contact number of attending clinician, if urgent antimicrobial therapy is required.
5. Report the suspected incident to infection control team.

Identifying a single, common source of infection (if there is one) requires the combined efforts of the infection control team, and other members of hospital staff. They will have to:
- take a close look at the epidemiology of the suspected outbreak.
- collect clinical and environmental specimens
- review clinical practice on the ward
- possibly wait for the results of molecular investigations.

It is important that preventive action taken on the basis of first impressions is not allowed to spoil these investigations.

## HOW TO CONTROL AN OUTBREAK

### PROCEDURE

1. Define the problem, as far as information allows.
2. Make sure presumptive therapy and diagnostic tests are ordered.
3. Consider the level of support needed: is this a major incident? Ask:
   - Are the lives of patients, staff or the community at risk?
   - Are these patients at risk of significant morbidity?
   - Is the continued provision of inpatient care under threat?

*Yes* The infection Control Committee should meet urgently to discuss action to be taken, and to set up an Action Team to include all other senior staff needed to ensure that control measures are applied quickly and efficiently.

*No* The Infection Control Team may be able to deal with the problem by forming an Incident Group to include other senior staff as required, e.g. representatives from the affected clinical services, occupational health and administration.

4. Introduce preliminary control measures.
5. Construct an information base to establish priorities for further interventions:
   - Using your outline problem definition, find as many cases as possible.
   - Search for possible connecting factors in the case notes, lab reports, ward, clinic and theatre records.
   - Review experience of similar outbreaks in the published literature.
6. Analyse the information you have collected:
   - Draw an epidemic curve (cases v. time).
   - Is the problem still active?
   - Chart possible risk factors for exposure or transmission.
   - If risk factors are unclear, consider case-control study.
   - Calculate probable exposure–infection intervals.
   - Outline likely source, transmission route and high risk groups.
7. Use continuing surveillance to assess impact of inital measures.
8. Do you need to introduce further interventions?

*Yes* Introduce measures appropriate to source, transmission route and high risk groups as outlined in 6 above; return to continued surveillance.

*No* Write up management of outbreak and report back to the Infection Control Committee, with recommendations for revised infection control policy, if indicated.

# REPORTING INFECTIONS FOR EPIDEMIOLOGICAL PURPOSES

## Priority organisms and infections

Some infections must be reported for epidemiological purposes. These are summarised in Table 4.7.

---

**TABLE 4.7    Priority organisms and infections**

**BACTERIAL**

Actinomyces

Aeromonas

*Bacillus anthracis*

*Bacillus cereus*

*Bordetella pertussis*

Borrelia

Brucella

Campylobacter

*Chlamydia pneumoniae*

*Chlamydia psittaci*

*Chlamydia trachomatis*

*Clostridium botulinum**

*Clostridium tetani* (clinical tetanus only)*

Clostridium, others (specify)

*Corynebacterium diphtheriae* (toxogenic and nontoxogenic)*

Erysipelothrix

Enteropathogenic *Escherichia coli*

Gas gangrene (by organism)

Group A streptococcus (invasive disease)

*Haemophilus influenzae* (invasive disease)*

Legionella*

Leptospira

Listeria*

Mycobacterium*

Mycoplasma

*Neisseria gonorrhoeae*

*Neisseria meningitidis* (not asymptomatic carriage)

Nocardia

Ophthalmia neonatorum (by organism)

Pasteurella

Plesiomonas

Salmonella*

Shigella

**TABLE 4.7  Priority organisms and infections (cont'd)**

*Streptobacillus moniliformis*

Vibrio

Yersinia

**FUNGI**

Absidia

Aspergillus

Blastomyces

Candida/Torulopsis

Coccidioides

Cryptococcus

Fusarium

Histoplasma

Paracoccidioides

*Penicillium marneffii*

Rhizomucor

Rhizopus

Scedosporum

Sporothrix

**HELMINTHS**

Diphyllobothrium

Dracunculus

Echinococcus

Fasciola

Hookworm

Filaria

Schistosoma

Strongyloides

Taenia

Trichuris

Toxocara

**PROTOZOA**

Acanthamoeba

Cryptosporidium

*Entamoeba histolytica*

*Giardia lamblia*

Hartmanella

Leishmania

Naegleria

Plasmodium (specify)

Pneumocystis

Toxoplasma

Trypanosoma

**TABLE 4.7    Priority organisms and infections (cont'd)**

**VIRAL AND OTHERS**

Adenovirus

Arbovirus

Astrovirus

Calicivirus

*Chlamydia psittaci*

*Chlamydia trachomatis*

Coronavirus

Cowpox

Coxiella

Coxsackie

Cytomegalovirus

EB virus (excluding uncomplicated glandular fever)

Echovirus

Hepatitis A, B*, C, E* Report should state whether infection is acute or chronic, with supporting laboratory results.

Herpes simplex (genital, neonatal, meningitis, encephalitis or deaths only)

HIV*

HTLV*

Influenza

Measles*

Molluscum contagiosum

Mumps*

Mycoplasma

Orf/paravaccinia

Papillomavirus

Papovavirus

Parainfluenza

Parvovirus B19*

Poliovirus

Polyomavirus

Rabies [Clinical and/or risk factor data desirable as part of report]

Reovirus

Respiratory syncytical virus

Rhinovirus

Rickettsia

Rotavirus

Rubella*

Small round structured virus (including Norwalk)

Varicella-zoster (neonatal, meningitis, encephalitis, pneumonia, pregnant cases or deaths only)

*Clinical and/or risk factor data desirable as part of report
Source: Public Health Laboratory Service; Communicable Diseases Surveillance Centre

## CORE SURVEILLANCE DATA

The following information is required on all reports for all organisms reported by every laboratory:

- source and reporting laboratory
- reference laboratory (where relevant)
- patient identification (laboratory accession number, soundex code, name, or GU clinic number)
- date of birth
- sex
- organism
- date of onset
- specimen type(s)
- specimen date(s)
- identification method(s) — not required if report is on CDR form 1, or identical format.

### Augmented surveillance data

Essential data for HIV, hepatitis A, B, C, and E, and salmonellas are:

- clinical features
- epidemiological features.

### Antimicrobial susceptibilities

Susceptibility test results are required with reports of systemic infections, apart from:

- fungi
- anaerobic bacteria
- opportunist mycobacteria
- coagulase negative staphylococci
- Gram positive bacilli.

### Reporting practice

Unless other arrangements have been agreed locally, reporting should be by the laboratory that received the specimen. Reports should be sent after completing identification procedures, except for Salmonellas (report after preliminary identification), the first time a given organism is identified for each patient. Report to the Communicable Disease Surveillance Centre (except Salmonellas, which should be reported to the Enteric Pathogens Laboratory, CPHL) on CDR forms, computer generated forms in CDR format or by electronic file transfer. (These reporting guidelines are reproduced with permission from the Public Health Laboratory Service, UK.)

# VARICELLA–ZOSTER IN HOSPITAL

The immunocompromised, newborns and pregnant mothers are all at increased risk of severe varicella infection, such as fulminant varicella pneumonia. Varicella-zoster immunoglobulin (VZIg) is available for contacts but is in short supply, and therefore has to be restricted to high risk contacts. VZIg does not prevent infection but should reduce its severity of infection.

## Procedure

- VZIg should be given as soon as possible after exposure, and within 4 days, though some benefit may be obtained up to 10 days after exposure.
- Infant dose: 250 mg.
- Adult dose: 1000 mg.

## Indications

Give VZIg in the following situations:

- Immune suppression, with no history of varicella or recent steroids.
- Bone marrow transplant, even if there has been previous varicella.
- Neonates
  — if maternal varicella 7 days before to 1 month after delivery
  — if seronegative mother and any varicella contact
  — if < 1 kg or < 30/40 and any varicella contact.
- Pregnant women who are seronegative and have had any varicella contact.

Varicella contacts must be checked for past history of chickenpox. If unknown or uncertain, they should be tested for VZ antibodies. VZIg is not required for people with pre-existing varicella infection or immunity.
  VZIg is of no use in treatment of chickenpox or shingles.

# ZOONOSIS RESERVOIRS

Zoonosis is a disease where animals are either a primary source or a major reservoir of infection. The various means of transmission are shown in Table 4.8.

**TABLE 4.8   Zoonosis: means of transmission**

| Disease | Source of infection |
|---|---|
| **Direct contact** | |
| Anthrax | Animal carcass, hide, hair, bones |
| Erysipeloid | Decaying organic matter; animals, fish |
| Fleas | Domestic animals, especially cats |
| Monkeypox | Chimpanzees, monkeys, squirrels |
| Orf | Sheep, goats |
| Ringworm | Various animals |
| Sarcoptic mange | Dogs, intimate contact |
| Vesicular stomatitis | Cows, pigs, horses |
| **Contact with organs, blood, body fluids** (e.g. raw offal or products of conception) | |
| Anthrax | Animal carcases, especially herbivores |
| Brucellosis | Genitourinary infection in cows, goats, sheep, pigs and other animals |
| Erysipeloid | Animals, fish |
| Glanders | Horses |
| Leptospirosis | Animal urine, especially dogs, rodents |
| Lymphocytic choriomeningitis | Rodents, especially hamsters, mice |
| Ornithosis (psittacosis) | Birds, especially parrots, budgies |
| *Pasteurella multocida* | Cats and dogs |
| Q fever | Cows, sheep, goats, other animals |
| **Contact with animal faeces** | |
| Creeping eruption (cutaneous larva migrans) | Dogs, cats |
| Tetanus | Many domestic and wild animals |
| **Faecal–oral transmission** | |
| Campylobacter | (*C. fetus*) cows, sheep |
| Cryptosporidiosis | Calves, lambs, other young animals |
| Giardiasis | Cats, dogs, wild animals (check in community outbreak) |
| Hepatitis A | Shellfish |
| Hydatid disease | Sheep, cows in close contact with dogs |

**TABLE 4.8   Zoonosis: means of transmission (cont'd)**

| | |
|---|---|
| Adenovirus | |
| Lymphocytic choriomeningitis | Rodents, especially hamsters, mice |
| Pentastomiasis | Lizard handling, snakes, undercooked meat |
| Salmonella | Chickens, reptiles, other domestic animals |
| Larva migrans (visceral/ocular) | Dogs, many other mammals, birds |
| Yersiniosis | Wild animals |
| **Respiratory transmission** | |
| Anthrax | Animal carcases, especially herbivores |
| Glanders | Horses |
| Lymphocytic choriomeningitis | Hamsters, other rodents |
| Ornithosis (psittacosis) | Parrots, budgies, other birds |
| Pasteurella multocida | Cats and dogs |
| Q fever | Cows, sheep, goats, pigs, other animals |
| Tuberculosis | Cows, other mammals |
| Tularaemia | Wild mammals, not in UK |
| **Bites and scratches** | |
| Cat scratch disease | Cats to dogs |
| DF-2 | Dogs |
| Lymphocytic choriomeningitis | Hamsters, other rodents |
| Pasteurella multocida | Cats and dogs |
| Rabies | Dogs, bats, foxes, raccoons, other animals |
| Rat bite fever | Rats, other rodents, cats, dogs, pigs, squirrels |
| Tularaemia | Wild mammals, not in UK |

# REFERENCE SOURCES

# CENTRES OF EXCELLENCE

## REFERENCE LABORATORIES: UK

**Centre for Applied Microbiological Research,** Porton Down, Salisbury, Wiltshire, SP4 0JG
Phone: 01980–612100; fax: 01980–611096 (general)
Phone: 01980–612453; fax: 01980–612731 (special pathogens, arboviruses and rickettsiae)

**Entomological Department, Natural History Museum**, London SW7 5BD
Phone: 0171–938–9462
**Entomological Medical Reference Centre, Department of Medical Parasitology, London School of Tropical Medicine**, Keppel Street, London, WC1E 7HT
Phone: 0171–927–2351

**PHLS (Public Health Laboratory Service**). Central Public Health Laboratory, 61 Colindale Avenue, London, NW9 5HT
Phone: 0181–200–4400; fax: 0181–200–7874
Specialist units:
- Food Enteric Division
- Hospital and Respiratory Infection Division
- Nosocomial Infection Surveillance Unit
- National Collection of Type Cultures
- Scientific Support Services Division
- Virus Reference Division
- PHLS Anaerobe Reference Unit, Department of Medical Microbiology and PHL, University Hospital Wales, Heath Park, Cardiff CF4 4XW
  Phone: 01222-742378; fax: 01222-744123
- PHLS Brucella Reference Unit PHL, St Mary's General Hospital, East Wing, Milton Road, Portsmith, Hants PO3 6AQ
  Phone: 01705-866202; fax: 01705-824652
- PHLS Communicable Disease Surveillance Centre (CDSC), 61 Colindale Avenue, London, NW9 5EQ
  Phone: +44 (0)181 200 6868; fax: +44 (0)181 200 7868
  Website: http://www.open.gov.uk/cdsc/cdschome.htm
  Divisions:
  –Environmental Surveillance Unit
  –Epidemiology (respiratory, enteric, nosocomial, zoonotic infections)
  –Immunisation
  –PHLS AIDS and STD Centre
  –Regional Services
  –Support Services
  –Statistics Unit

- PHLS Antiviral Susceptibility Reference Unit, PHL, Birmingham Heartlands Hospital, Bordesley Green East, Birmingham B9 5SS
  Phone: 0121 766 6611, ext: 4987; fax: 0121 772 6229
- PHLS Crytosporidium Reference Unit, PHL, Ysbyty Glan Clwyd, Rhyl, Denbighshire LL18 5UJ
  Phone: 01745 583737, ext: 4556; fax: 01745 584179
- PHLS Food Microbiology Research Unit, PHL, Church Lane, Heavitree, Exeter EX2 5AD
  Phone: 01392 402953; fax: 01392 412835
- PHLS Genitourinary Infection Reference Laboratory, PHL, Myrtle Road, Kingsdown, Bristol BS2 8EL
  Phone: 0117 929 1326; fax: 0117 922 6611
- PHLS *H. Influenzae* Reference Unit, PHL, Level 6/7 John Radcliffe Hospital, Headington, Oxford OX3 9DH
  Phone: 018365 220862; fax: 01703 220890
- PHLS Leptospria Reference Laboratory, PHL, County Hospital, Hereford HR1 2ER
  Phone: 01432 277707; fax: 01432 351369
- PHLS Lyme Disease Reference Unit, PHL, Level B, South Block, SGH, Southampton SO16 6YD
  Phone: 01703 794810; fax: 01703 774316
- PHLS Malaria Reference Laboratory, London School of Hygiene and Tropical Medicine, Keppel Street, London WC1E 7HT
  Phone: 0171 927 2437; fax: 0171 637 0248
- PHLS Meningococcal Reference Unit, PHL, Withington Hospital, Manchester M20 2LR
  Phone: 0161 291 4628; fax: 0161 446 2180
- PHLS Mycobacterium Reference Unit, PHL and Medical Microbiology, King's College School of Medicine and Dentistry, King's College Hospital, East Dulwich Grove, London SE22 8QF
  Phone: 0181 693 2830; fax: 0171 346 6477
- PHLS Mycology Reference Laboratory, Bristol PHL, Myrtle Road, Kingsdown, Bristol BS2 8EL
  Phone: 0117 928 5028; fax: 0117 922 6611
- PHLS Parasitology Reference Laboratory, Department of Clinical Parasitology, Hospital for Tropical Diseases, 4 St Pancras Way, London NW1 0PE
  Phone: 0171 530 3450; fax: 0171 383 0041
- PHLS Seroepidemiology Unit, PHL, Royal Preston Hospital, P.O. Box 202, Sharoe Green Lane, Preston PR2 9HG
  Phone: 01772 710114; fax: 01772 710166
- PHLS Toxoplasma Reference Unit, PHL, Singleton Hospital, Sgeth, Abertawe, Swansea SA2 8QA
  Phone: 01792 205666, ext: 5058; fax: 01792 202320

- PHLS Water and Environmental Microbiology Research Unit, PHL, University Hospital, Queens Medical Centre, Nottingham NG7 2UH
Phone: 0115 970 9163, ext: 44942; fax: 0115 942 2190

## INTERNATIONAL REFERENCE CENTRES

**Australasian College of Tropical Medicine**
ACTM Secretariat, Anton Breinl Centre, James Cook University, Townsville, Queensland 4811, Australia
Phone: +61 077 21 2281; fax: +61 077 71 5032

**Institut Pasteur**
28 rue du Docteur Roux, Cedex 15, F-75724 Paris, France
Phone: (01133) 145 68 80 00; fax: (01133) 40 61 30 30
Website: Homepage http://web.pasteur.fr/welcome-uk.html

**Institute of Tropical Medicine, Nagasaki**
ITM, Nagasaki University, 1–12–4 Sakamoto, Nagasaki 852, Japan
Phone: 0958 49 7820; fax: 0958 49 7821
Website: http://133.45.224.19/

**National Center for Infectious Diseases, Centers for Disease Control and Prevention (CDC),**
1600 Clifton Road, mailstop C-12, Atlanta GA 30333, USA
Phone: +1 (404) 639 3311
Website: http://www.cdc.gov/ncidod/ncid.htm

**World Health Organisation (WHO)**
CH-1211 Geneva 27, Switzerland
Phone: +41 22 791 2111; fax: +41 22 791 0746
E-mail: postmaster@who.ch
Website: http://www.who.ch
Offices:
- Africa
P.O. Box no. 6, Brazzaville, Congo
Phone: +242 83 38 60 or 64; fax: +242 83 9400
E-mail: afro@who.org
- Americas (PAHO)
525, 23rd Street, NW, Washington, D.C. 20037, USA
Phone: +1 202 861 3200; fax: +1 202 223 5971
E-mail: postmaster@paho.org
- Eastern Mediterranean
P.O. Box 1517, Alexandria, 21511, Egypt
Phone: +203 48 202 23 or 24; fax: +203 48 38 9 16
E-mail: postmaster@who.sci.eg

- Europe
  8 Scherfigsvej, DK-2100, Copenhagen 0, Denmark
  Phone: +45 39 17 17 17; fax: +45 39 17 18 18
  E-mail: postmaster@who.dk
- Southeast Asia
  World Health House, Indrapratha Estate, Mahatma Ghandi Road, New Delhi 110002, India
  Phone: +91 11 331 7804 or 7823; fax: +91 11 331 8607 or 7972
  E-mail: postmaster@who.ernet.in
- Western Pacific
  P.O. Box 2932, 1099 Manila, Philippines
  Phone: +632 521 84 21; fax: + 632 52 11 036
  E-mail: postmaster@who.org.ph

**India:** Department of Microbiology, All India Institute of Medical Sciences, Ansari Nagar, New Delhi 110 029, India
Website: http://www.pugmorks.com/aiims

**Malaysia:** Institute for Medical Research, Jalan Pahang. 50588 Kuala Lumpur, Malaysia
Phone: +603 298 6033; fax: +603 292 0675

**Philippines:** Tropical Disease Research Foundation, Makati Medical Center, Makati, Metro Manila, Philippines
Website: http://www.sequel.net/~mmcphi/menu99.htm

**Thailand:** Faculty of Tropical Medicine, Mahidol University, 420/6 Rajvithi Road, Bangkok 10400

# JOURNALS

## GENERAL

**British Medical Journal**
BMA House, Tavistock Square, London, WC1H 9JR
Classified (jobs) website: http://www.bmj.com/bmj
Guidelines to authors: 1st issue in January each year

**The Lancet**
42 Bedford Square, London, WC1B 3SL, UK
Phone: +44 (0)171 436 4981; fax: +44 (0)171 436 7550
E-mail: lanceteditorial@elsevier.co.uk
Website: http://www.thelancet.com
Guidelines to authors: 1st issue each month, after letters

**New England Journal of Medicine:**
The editor, NEJM, 10 Shattuck Street, Boston, MA 02115–6094, USA
E-mail (submitted publication status): status@edit.nejm.org
Website: http://www.nejm.org
Instructions to authors: listed in contents on front cover every issue

## GENERAL PATHOLOGY

**Journal of Clinical Pathology**
The editors, BMA House, Tavistock Square, London, WC1H 9JR
Instructions to authors on worldwide web:
Website: http://neuronott.nottingham.ac.uk/WEBpages/pathology/tocs/jepath.htm

**Pathology**
Editorial Office, Royal College of Pathologists of Australasia:
Durham Hall, 207, Albion Street, Surry Hills, NSW 2020, Australia
Phone: +61 (02) 332 4266; fax: +61 (02) 380 5948
Instructions for contributors: every issue on inside of back cover

## MICROBIOLOGY AND INFECTION

**Antimicrobial Agents and Chemotherapy**
Publications office, American Society for Microbiology, 1325 Massachussetts
Ave NW, Washington, D.C. 20005–4171, USA
Phone: +1 202 737 3600; fax: +1 202 942 9346
Website: http//www.asmusa.org/jnlsrc/acc1.htm
Instructions to authors: January edition every year, reprints available from
Publications office

## Clinical Microbiology and Infection
Editorial office, Université Paris VI, 15 Rue de l'École de Médecine, 75270 Paris Cedex 06, France
Phone: +331 43 25 12 82; fax: 331 43 25 12 54
Guidelines to authors: 1st issue each volume, towards end of journal

## Communicable Disease Report (CDR)
Editor, PHLS Communicable Disease Surveillance Centre, 61 Colindale Avenue, London, NW9 5EQ
Phone: +44 (0)181 200 6868; fax: +44 (0) 181 200 7868

## Emerging Infectious Diseases (on-line journal)
National Center for Infectious Diseases, Centers for Disease Control and Prevention (CDC), 1600 Clifton Road, mailstop C-12, Atlanta GA 30333, USA
Phone: +1 404 639 3967; fax: +1 404 639 3039
E-mail: eideditor@cidodl.em.cdc.gov
Website: http://www.cdc.gov/neidod/EID/eidtext.htm

## Journal of Antimicrobial Chemotherapy
Editor-in-chief, JAC Editorial Office, 11, the Wharf, Bridge Street, Birmingham, B1 2JS, UK
Phone: +44 (0)121 633 0415; fax: +44 (0)121 643 9497
E-mail: 100441.2540@compuserve.com
Note to contributors: every issue, and website:
http://www.hbuk.co.uk/wbs/jac/i2author.htm

## Journal of Clinical Microbiology
Publications office, American Society for Microbiology, 1325 Massachussetts Ave NW, Washington, D.C. 20005–4171, USA
Phone: +1 202 737 3600; fax: +1 202 942 9346
Website: http://asmua.edoc.com/jcm
Instructions to authors: January edition every year, reprints available from publications office

## Journal of Hospital Infection
Editor, Department of Microbiology, UMDS, 4th Floor, Tower Block, Guy's Hospital, London Bridge, London, SE1 9RT
Phone: +44 (0)171 955 8871; fax: +44 (0)171 955 8853
Website: http://www.hbuk.co.uk/wbs/jhi
Note to contributors: inside cover most issues

## Transactions of the Royal Society for Tropical Medicine and Hygiene
Editorial office, Royal Society of Tropical Medicine and Hygiene, Manson House, 26 Portland Place, London, W1N 4EY
Phone: +44 (0)171 580 2127; fax: +44 (0)171 436 1387
Notice to contributors: inside front cover every issue; details given towards end of 1st issue of each volume

**WHO Weekly Epidemiological Record**
World Health Organisation headquarters, CH-1211 Geneva 27, Switzerland
Phone: +41 22 791 2111; fax: +41 22 791 0746
E-mail: postmaster@who.ch
Website: http://www.who.ch/wer/wer_home.htm

# ORGANISATIONS

**American Society for Microbiology**
1325 Massachussetts Ave NW, Washington, D.C. 20005–4171, USA
Phone: +1 202 737 3600; fax: +1 202 942 9346
Website: http://www.asmusa.org/asm.htm

**Association of Medical Microbiologists**
Dr EP Wright, Department of Microbiology, Conquest Hospital, The Ridge,
St Leonards-on-Sea, East Sussex, TN 37 7RD, UK

**Australian Society for Microbiology**
Unit 23, 20 Commercial Road, Melbourne, Victoria 3004, Australia
Phone: +61 3 9867 8699; fax: +61 3 9867 8722
E-mail: contact by phone for details
Website: http://www.vicnet.net.au/~asm/welcome.htm

**British Society for Antimicrobial Chemotherapy**
Information about the society may be found in the current edition of the
Journal of Antimicrobial Chemotherapy (q.v.)

**European Society of Clinical Microbiology and Infectious Diseases**
P.O. Box 11 31, D-82018, Taufkirchen, Germany
Phone: +49 89 612 81 76; fax: +49 89 612 61 62

**Infection Control Nurses Association (UK)**
Information about the association can be found in the current edition of the
Infection Control Journal, supplied as a supplement to the Nursing Times
every two months

**Hospital Infection Society**
Information about the society can be obtained from the current edition of the
Journal of Hospital Infection (q.v.)

**Pathology Society of Great Britain and Ireland**
2 Carlton House Terrace, London SW1Y 5AF, UK
Phone: +44 (0)171 976 1260; fax: +44 (0)171 976 1267

**Royal College of Pathologists of Australasia**
Durham Hall, 207, Albion Street, Surry Hills, NSW 2020, Australia
Phone: +61 (02) 332 4266; fax: +61 (02) 380 5948

**Royal College of Pathologists (UK)**
2 Carlton House Terrace, London, SW1Y 5AF
Phone: +44 (0)171 930 5861; fax: +44 321 0523

**Royal Society of Tropical Medicine and Hygiene**
Manson House, 26 Portland Place, London, W1N 4EY
Phone: +44 (0)171 580 2127; fax: +44 (0)171 436 1387

## TRAVEL HEALTH ADVICE

General advice in the UK can be found in the Department of Health booklet, *Health Advice for Travellers*, which is available free-of-charge in Post Offices. Most enquiries from the general public concerning prevention of travel-related infection and maintenance of health overseas should be passed on to a general practitioner or a travel health clinic.

Up-to-date epidemiological advice can be obtained via the WHO or CDC homepage on Worldwide Web (see below), and WHO have published a detailed guide on vaccinations and travel health, entitled, *International Travel and Health* (ISBN 92 4 158020 8).

You can obtain further advice from the Travel Unit at CDSC, phone: 0181–200–6868; or (if it concerns acute patient management) from the duty doctor at the London Hospital for Tropical Diseases, phone: 0171–387–4411.

Malaria prophylaxis is a complex issue, particularly as new and established forms of resistance are becoming common at the same time as travel to exotic tropical destinations becomes more popular. Remember:

- Chemoprophylaxis does not provide 100% protection.
- Travellers still need to avoid mosquito bites.
- They should continue taking tablets for 4 weeks after returning.
- Malaria may still occur several months after the return.

### TRAVEL MEDICINE ON THE WEB

Internet/worldwide web home pages:

1. Links to key websites (site design by David O Freedman MD, UAB)
   http://medinfo.dom.uab.edu/geomed/links.html
2. CDC travel information
   http://www.cdc.gov/travel/travel.html
3. Medical Advisory Service for Travellers Abroad (MASTA)
   http://dspace.dial.pipox.com/musta/index.html
4. WHO Weekly Epidemiological Record on-line
   http://www.who.ch/wer/wer_home.htm

# INDEX

# DIRECTORY

## HOSPITAL DEPARTMENTS

Department ................................................................................................
Extension ................................................................................................

Department ................................................................................................
Extension ................................................................................................

Department ................................................................................................
Extension ................................................................................................

Department ................................................................................................
Extension ................................................................................................

Department ................................................................................................
Extension ................................................................................................

Department ................................................................................................
Extension ................................................................................................

Department ................................................................................................
Extension ................................................................................................

Department ................................................................................................
Extension ................................................................................................

Department ................................................................................................
Extension ................................................................................................

Department ................................................................................................
Extension ................................................................................................

Department ................................................................................................
Extension ................................................................................................

Department ................................................................................................
Extension ................................................................................................

Department ................................................................................................
Extension ................................................................................................

Department ................................................................................................
Extension ................................................................................................

Department ................................................................................................
Extension ................................................................................................

Department ................................................................................................
Extension ................................................................................................

# HOSPITAL CONTACTS

Name .......................................................................................................................
Department ...............................................................................................................
Extension .................................................................................................................
Pager .......................................................................................................................

Name .......................................................................................................................
Department ...............................................................................................................
Extension .................................................................................................................
Pager .......................................................................................................................

Name .......................................................................................................................
Department ...............................................................................................................
Extension .................................................................................................................
Pager .......................................................................................................................

Name .......................................................................................................................
Department ...............................................................................................................
Extension .................................................................................................................
Pager .......................................................................................................................

Name .......................................................................................................................
Department ...............................................................................................................
Extension .................................................................................................................
Pager .......................................................................................................................

Name .......................................................................................................................
Department ...............................................................................................................
Extension .................................................................................................................
Pager .......................................................................................................................

Name .......................................................................................................................
Department ...............................................................................................................
Extension .................................................................................................................
Pager .......................................................................................................................

Name .......................................................................................................................
Department ...............................................................................................................
Extension .................................................................................................................
Pager .......................................................................................................................

Name .......................................................................................................................
Department ...............................................................................................................
Extension .................................................................................................................
Pager .......................................................................................................................

## GENERAL PRACTITIONERS

Name ...............................................................................................................
Address ...............................................................................................................
Phone/fax ...............................................................................................................
E-mail ...............................................................................................................

Name ...............................................................................................................
Address ...............................................................................................................
Phone/fax ...............................................................................................................
E-mail ...............................................................................................................

Name ...............................................................................................................
Address ...............................................................................................................
Phone/fax ...............................................................................................................
E-mail ...............................................................................................................

Name ...............................................................................................................
Address ...............................................................................................................
Phone/fax ...............................................................................................................
E-mail ...............................................................................................................

Name ...............................................................................................................
Address ...............................................................................................................
Phone/fax ...............................................................................................................
E-mail ...............................................................................................................

Name ...............................................................................................................
Address ...............................................................................................................
Phone/fax ...............................................................................................................
E-mail ...............................................................................................................

Name ...............................................................................................................
Address ...............................................................................................................
Phone/fax ...............................................................................................................
E-mail ...............................................................................................................

Name ...............................................................................................................
Address ...............................................................................................................
Phone/fax ...............................................................................................................
E-mail ...............................................................................................................

Name ...............................................................................................................
Address ...............................................................................................................
Phone/fax ...............................................................................................................
E-mail ...............................................................................................................

# SUPPLIERS AND OTHER CONTACTS

Name .........................................................................................................
Address .........................................................................................................
Phone/fax .........................................................................................................
E-mail .........................................................................................................

Name .........................................................................................................
Address .........................................................................................................
Phone/fax .........................................................................................................
E-mail .........................................................................................................

Name .........................................................................................................
Address .........................................................................................................
Phone/fax .........................................................................................................
E-mail .........................................................................................................

Name .........................................................................................................
Address .........................................................................................................
Phone/fax .........................................................................................................
E-mail .........................................................................................................

Name .........................................................................................................
Address .........................................................................................................
Phone/fax .........................................................................................................
E-mail .........................................................................................................

Name .........................................................................................................
Address .........................................................................................................
Phone/fax .........................................................................................................
E-mail .........................................................................................................

Name .........................................................................................................
Address .........................................................................................................
Phone/fax .........................................................................................................
E-mail .........................................................................................................

Name .........................................................................................................
Address .........................................................................................................
Phone/fax .........................................................................................................
E-mail .........................................................................................................

Name .........................................................................................................
Address .........................................................................................................
Phone/fax .........................................................................................................
E-mail .........................................................................................................